SECOND EDITION

STRENGTH TRAINING

by the experts

Daniel P. Riley

Strength Coach
Washington Redskins

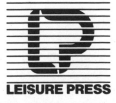

LEISURE PRESS

CHAMPAIGN, ILLINOIS

Published by Leisure Press
A division of Human Kinetics Publishers, Inc.
Box 5076
Champaign, IL 61820

Library of Congress Catalog Card No. 81-85627
ISBN 0-88011-041-4

Front cover photo: John Dotson
Back cover artwork: Lanny Somese

CONTENTS

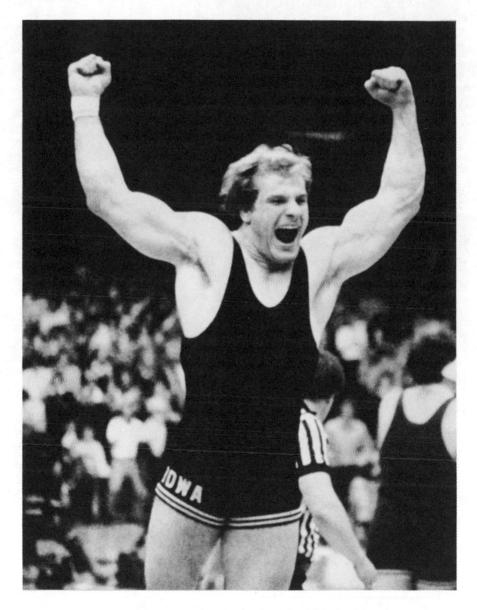

A stronger athlete is a better (and healthier) athlete.

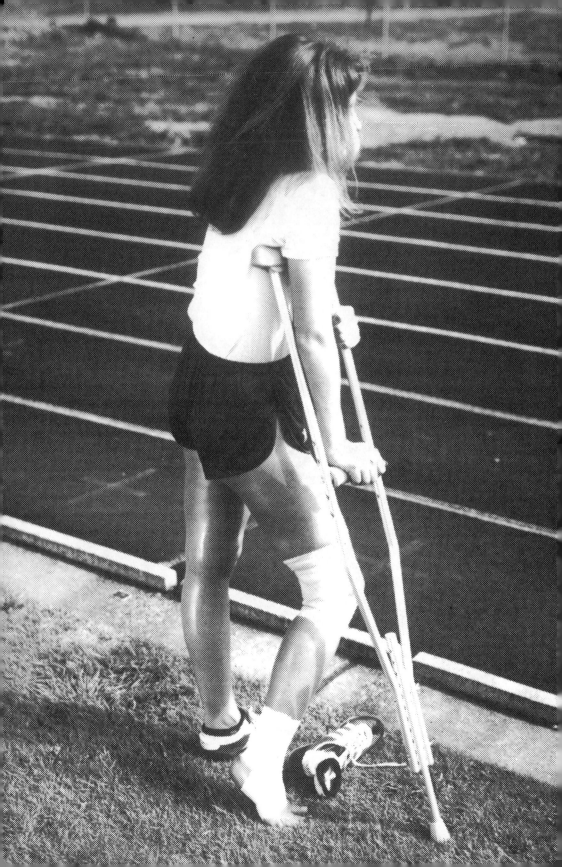

1

STRENGTH TRAINING: HEALTH INSURANCE FOR THE ATHLETE

by
James A. Peterson, Ph.D.
Director of Sports Medicine
Women's Sports Foundation

...Strength training will bind athletes and make them muscle-bound.
...Higher levels of strength and endurance will impair an athlete's motor skills.
...Individuals have no need for muscular fitness above their "God-given" levels.
...Lifting weights will only turn an individual into a miniature Arnold Schwartzenegger clone.

What do the above statements have in common? Two things. First they're among the more popular reasons advanced by both coaches and athletes for their failure to either implement or engage in a strength training program; and second, they're all totally FALSE.

All athletes have a great need for a high level of muscular fitness. Regretably, many individuals view strength training as a form of torture so foreign to their personal needs and lifestyles that they would do almost anything to avoid it. Athletes in almost all sports are quick to point out successful athletes in their sport who never lifted weight #1 in their lives. Coupled with the seemingly never-ending list of groundless superstitions and practices attendant to strength training, these athletes continue to avoid any semblance of a strength training program. Given a diverse combination of skill, good fortune, and genetic "tickets," some of these individuals may even achieve a notable level of success within the athletic arena.

Although this article is directed at athletes and coaches, physically active, non-athlete readers can certainly apply the points discussed to their own situation.

What many athletes and coaches fail to realize, however, is that the athlete who has never lifted weights who is successful is successful NOT because he/she didn't lift weights, but IN SPITE OF IT. How many might-have-been Ted Williams or could-have-been Dick Butkus' were injured playing their sport and never had a chance to excel? Obviously, if a currently successful athlete who scoffs at the necessity for high levels of muscular fitness had been seriously injured earlier in his/her career, it is very likely that no one ever would have heard of him/her either.

The point behind the aforementioned discussion on injuries is the real basis for justifying the time and effort involved with strength training—TO REDUCE THE CHANCES OF INJURIES. You can be a great coach with great athletes who believe in you and respect you, but it simply won't be worth a tinker's damn (relatively speaking) if one of your kids is injured.

In 1974, while I was a member of the faculty at the United States Military Academy, USMA and Nautilus Sports/Medical Industries cosponsored a comprehensive study which investigated the interrelationship between selected fitness components and numerous strength training variables. During the course of that study, several physicians noted for their expertise in sports medicine visited West Point to view the study in progress. The list of individuals who spent several days at the Academy reads like a who's who (at the time) of renowned practitioners in sports medicine: Drs. Fred Allman, Fred Jackson, Jim Key, Robert Nirschel, and many others. To a man, these individuals expounded on the beneficial effect that higher levels of muscular fitness would have on reducing the incidence of athletic-related injuries. Their overwhelming, unanimous opinion: MORE THAN HALF THE INJURIES IN SPORTS COULD EASILY BE PREVENTED THROUGH PROPER STRENGTH TRAINING.

Given the fact that considerable research and pragmatic observations on campuses across the country have demonstrated (conclusively, I believe) that a properly conducted strength training program requires a MAXIMUM expenditure of 20-25 minutes, three times a week, what cheaper form of health insurance could possibly be obtained? To put it bluntly to the non-believer coaches, unless you have some personal covenant with God which guarantees that your athletes will not be injured, you have a LOT to gain from strength training. A coach's commitment to his kids, to his programs, and to himself simply shouldn't let him take the chance. Even if a single injury were prevented from having your team engage in a strength training program, the effort would be well worthwhile.

Another benefit of proper strength training is the positive effect that it will have on the performance capabilities of your athletes. Contrary to the popular misconception that strength training will somehow foul up or diminish the skills of your players, it will actually improve those skills and will increase the capacity of your athletes to perform those skills at a relatively high level for a longer period of time. Given the fact that every basic motor ability (one of the most critical factors affecting athletic performance)—agility, coordination, quickness, reaction time, power, balance, etc.—is influenced to some degree by an athlete's level of muscular fitness, it only stands to reason that properly developed, higher levels of muscular fitness will IMPROVE an athlete's motor skills. So as not to raise your hopes too high, however, strength training cannot turn a motor-moron-donkey into a veritable Man-of-War. Genetically speaking, God favors some athletes with more neurological "tickets" than others. For example, some individuals are born with natural quickness, while others are burdened by snail-like reactions—reactions that cannot be substantially improved by strength training.

Given the real value of higher levels of muscular fitness as a form of health insurance and the potential value of strength training on physical performance, I can only hope that sometime in the near future you will institute a strength training program for your athletes (if you don't already have one). Morally speaking, you're obligated. Pragmatically speaking, you'd be foolish if you didn't.

As you endeavor to channel your commitment to preventing injuries from afflicting your athletes, don't permit yourself to be sidetracked by the proverbial "3 Don'ts" of coaching.

DON'T #1: Don't let the lack of facilities or equipment discourage you. If necessary, juryrig an alternative. Unfortunately, but realistically, at any given time not everyone can afford to purchase the best strength training equipment. In these instances, alternative forms of resistance exercises (e.g., buddy training) will suffice.

DON'T #2: Don't let the perceived lack of time to implement a strength training program into your overall schedule thwart your efforts to institute such a program. What good are two hours of daily practice of fundamentals if your best player pulls a hamstring?

And finally, DON'T #3: Don't let the natural skepticism of your athletes towards the usefulness of strength training deter you from your efforts to make your athletes "as good as they can be." Without a high level of muscular fitness—a level which can only be achieved by engaging in a properly developed strength training program—they'll NEVER be as good as they can be. As a coach, you have the inherent privilege and somewhat awesome responsibility of helping your athletes take care of their most important personal possession—their healthy bodies. Strength training can help you in this task.

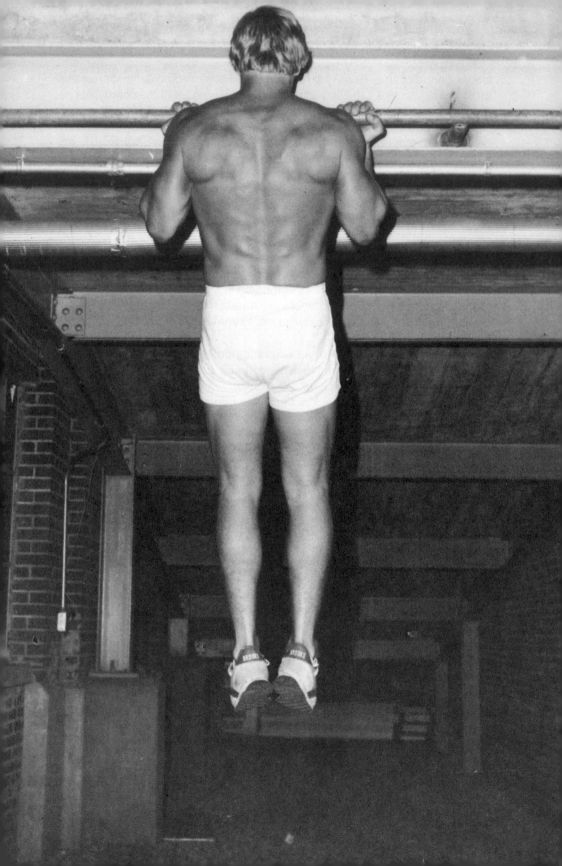

2

MUSCLES: PHYSIOLOGY AND FUNCTION

by
Daniel P. Riley
Washington Redskins

MUSCULAR PHYSIOLOGY

The human body is a system of levers with the force to move these levers being supplied by the muscles. A muscle is a mass of stored chemical energy which, when activated, will produce movement of the bones about their axis of rotation. Muscles that provide movement of the bones are called skeletal muscles. These muscles are composed of water (75%), proteins (20%), and inorganic salts (5%).

Scientists have concluded that the number of muscle fibers in a person's muscle group probably is established after the embryo has reached the age of 4 to 5 months. This means that when the strength and mass of a muscle is increased, the number of muscle fibers remains the same. The increase in size and strength of the muscle takes place by increasing the cross-sectional width of the existing muscle fibers.

Cross-sectional width.

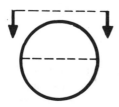

Individual muscle fiber before engaging in a strength development program

Cross-sectional width.

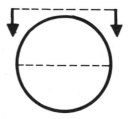

Individual muscle fiber after an increase in strength and muscle mass

11

Since new fibers cannot be added it should be obvious that the more muscle fibers you are born with, the greater will be your potential for gaining muscle strength and mass.

Muscle Structure

A muscle is composed of thousands of individual muscle fibers. If a muscle were bisected, it would resemble Figure 2-1. Muscles attach to bones by tendons. Do not confuse the function of a tendon with that of a ligament. A ligament attaches a bone to a bone while the tendon secures the muscle to the bone. Figure 2-2 illustrates the biceps muscle being secured to the upper and lower arm by the tendon. A tendon is a tough fibrous tissue that is attached to both the bone and the muscle. A tendon is capable of withstanding tremendous amounts of force placed upon it during a forceful contraction of the muscle. If a muscle itself were secured to the bone, it would surely be torn away from it during a forceful contraction.

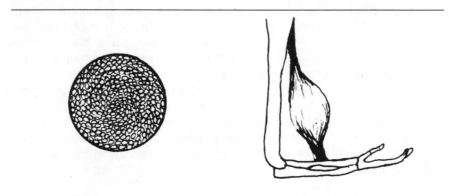

Figure 2-1   **Figure 2-2**

Muscle Fiber Recruitment

Throughout the entire muscle are thousands of motor units. The function of a motor unit is to receive messages via the central nervous system (CNS). The motor unit then releases a signal to a group of muscle fibers which forces them to contract.

A skeletal muscle will contract voluntarily or involuntarily when the CNS receives a signal from the various receptors of the body (brain, ears, eyes,·

touch). The CNS then transmits a signal to the motor unit which forces the muscle to contract.

Each individual motor unit is attached to several hundred muscle fibers. When a particular motor unit is fired (receives a message via the CNS), all of the muscle fibers attached to the motor unit will contract. This is known as the "all or nothing principle."

The greater the number of motor units you can recruit, the greater the number of muscle fibers you will have available for exercise. The recruitment of muscle fibers via the CNS is known as neuromuscular efficiency. A successful weight lifter or athlete must have a very high neuromuscular efficiency. The number of motor units recruited by the CNS will depend upon the task involved and the efficiency of your neuromuscular system. During an all-out effort in which you attempt to lift as much weight as you possibly can, you may only recruit from 30%-35% of all the muscle fibers you have available. To recruit all of the muscle fibers you have available, you should try to find a weight which will cause you to fail between 8 and 12 repetitions. The muscle fibers initially recruited will gradually fatigue which forces the CNS to constantly recruit new muscle fibers that have not yet been used. For maximum fiber recruitment, the muscle must exert an all-out effort while being unable to overcome the resistance somewhere between 8 and 12 repetitions.

Figure 2-3 illustrates how the neuromuscular system operates to recruit muscle fibers.

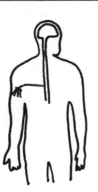

The brain receives a message and transmits the message to the CNS, the CNS then transmits this message to a nerve which relays the message to a motor unit which "fires" and forces all its muscle fibers to contract.

Figure 2-3.

Muscle Contraction

At present, the most widely accepted theory of a muscle fiber contracting is the sliding filament theory. Imagine that there are two filaments in each individual muscle fiber (Figure 2-4). When a fiber receives a signal from a motor unit to contract, the two filaments pull toward each other and continue to pull while one filament slides over the other causing the fiber to shorten. Figure 2-5 illustrates the fiber before and after contraction. When a muscle contracts, the individual fibers are shortening. This is called a concentric contraction. As the fibers shorten, they pull on the bones they are attached to causing movement. The biceps muscle contracting concentrically is depicted in Figure 2-6. When a muscle lengthens while resisting a force, it is called an eccentric contraction. The movement in Figure 2-6 is simply reversed.

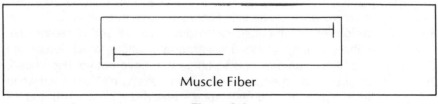

Muscle Fiber

Figure 2-4

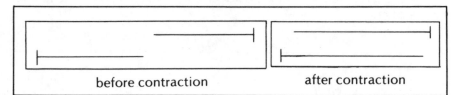

before contraction   after contraction

Figure 2-5

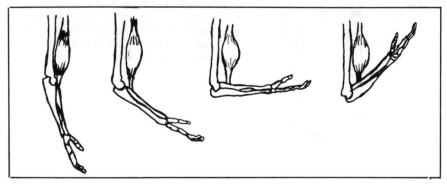

Figure 2-6

TYPES OF CONTRACTION

For discussion purposes, there are three different methods of exercise in which a muscle can be contracted: **isometrically, isotonically,** and **isokinetically.** An **isometric contraction** occurs when there is no movement of the levers involved while the length of the muscle remains constant. The resistance is immobilized at a fixed point during the range of movement of an exercise. When isometric training is utilized, it is recommended that a maximum effort be exerted for a period of 6-8 seconds.

Isometric training, however, has a few disadvantages:

- The strength is developed at one fixed position during a range of movement where there are many possible positions (Figure 2-7).
- It would be impossible to exercise all of these positions effectively utilizing isometric principles.
- The flexibility of the muscle will not be increased.
- There is no negative work accomplished.

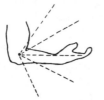

Isometrically, strength is developed only at one fixed position within a muscle's full range of movement.

Figure 2-7. An isometric contraction of the biceps.

An **isotonic contraction** occurs when a muscle lengthens and shortens through its full range of movement while lowering and raising a resistance. An isotonic contraction may be observed when a barbell is raised and lowered through a muscle's full range of movement.

An **isokinetic contraction** occurs when a muscle shortens while exerting a maximum effort throughout the muscle's entire range of movement. A piece of equipment designed to produce an isokinetic contraction is necessary for isokinetic training. The isokinetic machine mechanically regulates the speed of movement. This provides for a constant, maximum contraction throughout the entire range of movement while unaffecting the speed of movement.

Strength Curve

A muscle has different levels of strength varying or changing while moving through its particular range of movement. This variance in strength is due to the skeletal advantages and disadvantages which exist at different angles of the levels involved. As an arm or leg is raised, the angle at which the muscle is pulling on the bone changes. This angle determines the mechanical advantage or disadvantage. As the mechanical advantage increases, the muscle becomes capable of raising more weight. Obviously, as the mechanical advantage decreases, the muscle becomes capable of raising less weight. The point of the least mechanical advantage is often called the "sticking point" of an exercise. This is the point where the muscle will eventually fail and be unable to overcome the resistance.

Variable or Accommodating Resistance

Variable or accommodating resistance varies the resistance as a muscle contracts. This is designed to accommodate any changes in the strength of the muscle due to mechanical advantage and disadvantages (skeletal changes) occurring.

While performing an exercise with a barbell, the resistance remains constant throughout the entire range of movement. Therefore, a muscle is limited to the amount of weight it can overcome by the amount of weight it can lift at the muscle's least mechanical advantage. Maximum efficiency is obtained at only one point during a range of movement. Consequently, a muscle is limited to the amount of strength it can gain by the amount of weight it can overcome at its weakest point. This does not provide maximum muscle fiber recruitment at other points during the range of movement where a muscle is capable of lifting more weight. This limitation of the barbell brought about the introduction of equipment that varies the resistance to accommodate the strength curves of the muscles. These machines vary the resistance in order to obtain maximum muscle fiber recruitment throughout the entire range of movement.

Some isokinetic (e.g. CYBEX), Nautilus, and Universal machines are examples of machines which purport to provide accommodating resistance throughout the entire range of movement of an exercise. For example, when performing the bench press exercise, the mechanical advantage increases as your arms are extended. (The amount of weight you are capable of raising is much greater with the arms almost extended as compared to when the arms are flexed and the bar resting on your chest.)

The Universal bench press station, for example (Figure 2-8), has two sets of numbers on each of the weight plates. The lower number on the left represents the weight to be lifted in the starting position. The weight on the right side of the plate represents the amount of weight being lifted as your arms are almost extended. As your arms are extended, the weight gradually increases to accommodate the mechanical advantage of the muscles being used.

Varying resistance forces your body to recruit muscle fibers which would not have been recruited if the weight did not change through a muscle's range of movement. Consequently, the exercise becomes more efficient, thereby producing a greater increase in muscle mass and strength.

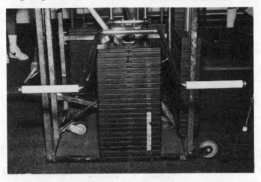

Figure 2-8

The Universal machine varies the resistance by the fulcrum of the movement arm as the weight is lifted. Figures 2-9 and 2-10 illustrate the changing position of the fulcrum of the movement arm on the Universal bench press as the arms are extended.

Nautilus machines vary the resistance through the use of a Nautilus cam. Figures 2-11 and 2-12 illustrate the changing position of the cam to accommodate the varying strength of the biceps.

Isokinetic machines often vary the resistance by the use of either a hydraulic clutch (Figure 2-13) or cylinders filled with fluid (Figure 2-14).

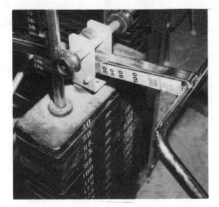

Figure 2-9

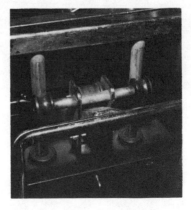

Figure 2-10

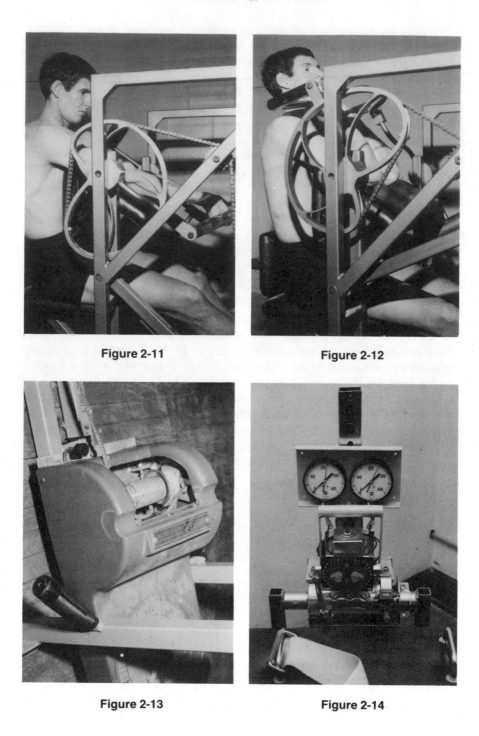

Figure 2-11

Figure 2-12

Figure 2-13

Figure 2-14

Muscle Soreness

Any new exercise performed at a moderately high level of intensity will cause localized soreness to the muscles involved. Although terms such as lactic acid or minute fiber tears have been used to explain this phenomenon, there is little agreement among the experts on the explanation of muscle soreness.

Many studies have been conducted which support the fact that the eccentric contraction (the lowering of the weight) causes the majority of soreness of an exercise. The lowering of the weight is the portion of the exercise in which the stretching of the muscle takes place.

Some experts feel that muscular soreness is evidently caused by a mechanical pull exerted by muscle fibers on intramuscular connective tissue. They conclude that since during negative work, muscle fibers lengthen and increase their tension, the number of participating fibers therefore decreases. The end result is a greater pull by each fiber in connective tissue, and local edema (swelling) gradually develops, causing pain.

Soreness after a new exercise may appear within a few hours. However, within 5 to 7 days, muscle soreness should gradually disappear if you continue to train every other day.

Muscle soreness can be minimized by gradually easing into the exercise program. It should be your goal to adapt to your program as quickly as possible. This will enable you to exert maximum efforts which in turn will stimulate the greatest gains in strength and muscle mass.

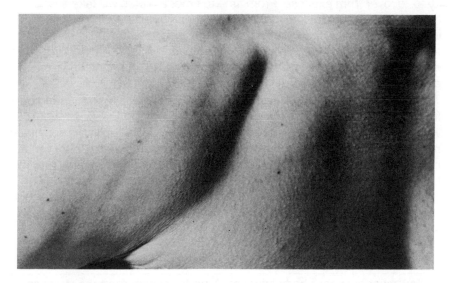

Muscle soreness can be minimized by gradually easing into the strength training program.

Adaptation Energy

The energy that allows your body to recover from exercise is called adaptation energy. This energy is used by your body whenever you expend energy. Walking to class, participating in athletics or physical education classes, and so on, deplete your body's supply of adaptation energy. This daily expenditure of energy is particularly difficult for an athlete. An athlete is left with very little adaptation energy to use to recover from a strength training workout. An athlete should, therefore, perform as few sets and exercises as are needed to stimulate the greatest increase in strength and muscle mass. High intensity workouts that are brief in nature will stimulate maximum gains in strength because they allow your body to totally recover from the demands placed on it.

Unfortunately, many coaches continue to associate the progress and success of an athlete with the quantity or amount of exercise he/she performs. They totally ignore an athlete's ability to recover from stressful activity.

An athlete can only perform so much exercise before he/she begins to reach a point of diminishing returns. A plateau or decrease in strength and performance will eventually be reached. A period of rest must follow which will provide the body the opportunity to replenish its supply of adaptation energy and recover from the large level of stress from which the body was unable to recover.

Many athletes, especially swimmers and runners, experience this inability to recover from exericse. From time to time, athletes will take a week or two off from training for one reason or another. Upon returning to their training schedule, they find that they have not only maintained their level of strength or fitness, but have actually increased their ability to perform. This can be attributed to their bodies finally "catching up" or recovering from the extensive stress.

Accordingly, you should realize that it is physiologically unsound to perform multiple sets of an exercise. An athlete, weightlifter, or bodybuilder who regularly performs 3-6 sets of an exercise, in all probability, is not totally recovering from the extensive demands of such a regimen. Better results could be obtained simply by decreasing the amount of exercises and the number of sets being performed.

Depletion of adaptation energy supply occurs when you have: too much exercise, inadequate time to recover between workouts, and inadequate sleep or diet.

You must give your body adequate time to recover from the stresses imposed upon it.

MUSCULAR FUNCTIONS

Most of the major muscle groups perform several functions. For example, the biceps rotate and flex the lower arm and raise the upper arm forward and upward. However, the primary function of the biceps is to flex the lower arm. It is hardly surprising, therefore, that it is difficult to remember and understand the many intricate movements that each muscle provides. Figures 2-15 and 2-16 provide an inclusive view of the musculature of the body.

Muscles of the Buttocks and Legs

● **Buttocks (Gluteals)**: The buttocks are primarily composed of three muscle groups: the gluteus maximus, gluteus medius, and gluteus minimus. The buttocks are the largest and strongest muscle group in the body. Their primary function is to extend the hip. They are the prime mover in activities similar to the vertical jump, barbell squat, sprinters start, etc. It is very difficult to isolate the buttocks muscles during exercise. The smaller and weaker muscles of the legs must assist to perform most exercises involving the buttocks. The buttocks can be effectively isolated when utilizing the Nautilus Hip and Back machines (refer to Chapter 13 for specific information).

● **Quadriceps**: The quadriceps are composed of four muscles which are located on the front side of the upper leg. Their primary function during exercise is to extend the leg (kicking motion from the knee). They assist in performing activities that involve running, jumping, and kicking. A primary exercise for the quadriceps is the leg extension.

● **Hamstrings**: The hamstrings are located on the backside of the upper leg. Their primary function is to flex the lower leg (raise the heel toward the buttocks). A primary exercise for the hamstrings is the leg curl. The hamstrings are very instrumental in sprinting.

● **Calves**: The calves are located on the backside of the lower leg. Their primary function is to allow you to elevate your heel off the floor. Any activity which involves the elevation of the heel off the floor will involve the calves. A primary exercise for the calves is the heel raise.

Muscles of the Torso (Back)

● **Latissimus Dorsi (Lats)**: The lats are located on your upper back. They can be palpated by reaching under the arm. Their primary function is to assist the biceps when performing a pulling movement. Some primary exercises for the lats are chinups, pullups, lat pulldowns, bentover rowing, swimming and rope climbing. Swimming and throwing movements involve the lats significantly.

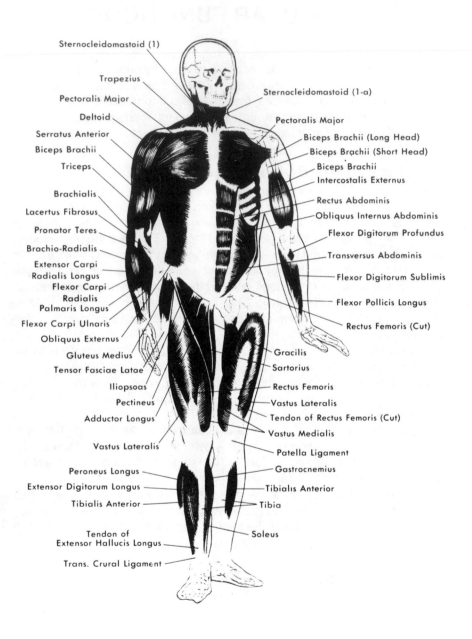

Sternocleidomastoid (1)
Trapezius
Pectoralis Major
Deltoid
Serratus Anterior
Biceps Brachii
Triceps
Brachialis
Lacertus Fibrosus
Pronator Teres
Brachio-Radialis
Extensor Carpi Radialis Longus
Flexor Carpi Radialis
Palmaris Longus
Flexor Carpi Ulnaris
Obliquus Externus
Gluteus Medius
Tensor Fasciae Latae
Iliopsoas
Pectineus
Adductor Longus
Vastus Lateralis
Peroneus Longus
Extensor Digitorum Longus
Tibialis Anterior
Tendon of Extensor Hallucis Longus
Trans. Crural Ligament

Sternocleidomastoid (1-a)
Pectoralis Major
Biceps Brachii (Long Head)
Biceps Brachii (Short Head)
Biceps Brachii
Intercostalis Externus
Rectus Abdominis
Obliquus Internus Abdominis
Flexor Digitorum Profundus
Transversus Abdominis
Flexor Digitorum Sublimis
Flexor Pollicis Longus
Rectus Femoris (Cut)
Gracilis
Sartorius
Rectus Femoris
Vastus Lateralis
Tendon of Rectus Femoris (Cut)
Vastus Medialis
Patella Ligament
Gastrocnemius
Tibialis Anterior
Tibia
Soleus

Figure 2-15. Anterior view of your muscles.

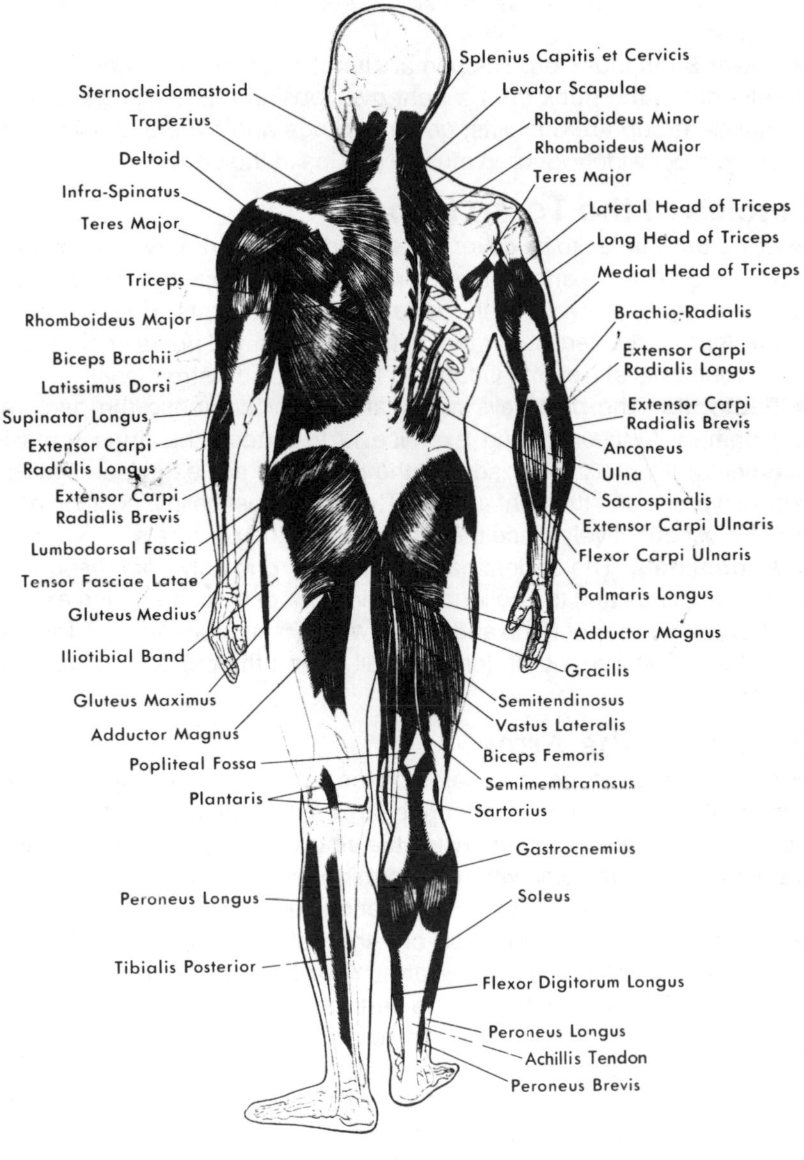

Sternocleidomastoid
Trapezius
Deltoid
Infra-Spinatus
Teres Major
Triceps
Rhomboideus Major
Biceps Brachii
Latissimus Dorsi
Supinator Longus
Extensor Carpi Radialis Longus
Extensor Carpi Radialis Brevis
Lumbodorsal Fascia
Tensor Fasciae Latae
Gluteus Medius
Iliotibial Band
Gluteus Maximus
Adductor Magnus
Popliteal Fossa
Plantaris
Peroneus Longus
Tibialis Posterior

Splenius Capitis et Cervicis
Levator Scapulae
Rhomboideus Minor
Rhomboideus Major
Teres Major
Lateral Head of Triceps
Long Head of Triceps
Medial Head of Triceps
Brachio-Radialis
Extensor Carpi Radialis Longus
Extensor Carpi Radialis Brevis
Anconeus
Ulna
Sacrospinàlis
Extensor Carpi Ulnaris
Flexor Carpi Ulnaris
Palmaris Longus
Adductor Magnus
Gracilis
Semitendinosus
Vastus Lateralis
Biceps Femoris
Semimembranosus
Sartorius
Gastrocnemius
Soleus
Flexor Digitorum Longus
Peroneus Longus
Achillis Tendon
Peroneus Brevis

Figure 2-16. Posterior view of your muscles.

● **Trapezius (Traps)**: The traps cover the upper portions of the back and neck. The primary function of the traps is to elevate your shoulder girdle (raise the shoulders upward). A primary exercise for the traps is the shoulder shrug. The trapezius muscle also protects the neck and shoulder girdle from injury.

● **Lower Back Muscles**: The primary function of the lower back muscles is to straighten the trunk from a bent over position. Exercises specific to this muscle group are deadlifts, goodmornings and hyperextensions. It is one of the most widely ignored muscle groups in the body.

Muscles of the Torso (Front)

● **Deltoids**: The deltoids cover the shoulder. The primary function of the deltoids is to raise the arms forward or sideward and upward. They also assist in movements involving the extension of the arms (pressing movements). A primary exercise for the deltoids is a seated press or side lateral raise (w/dumbbells) (refer to Chapter 11 for specific instructions).

● **Pectorals**: The pectoralis major and minor compose the pectorals. Their primary function during exercise is to extend the arms (pressing movements). Primary exercises for the pectorals are exercises similar to the bench press and the bent arm fly. The body must be in a position on the back to most effectively place the emphasis on the pectorals.

● **Abdominals**: The abdominal muscles are primarily composed of the rectus abdominus and the obliques. Their primary function during exercise is to stabilize and support the abdominal wall. The abdominals are forced to contract and stabilize the abdominal wall during the performance of most exercises.

Muscles of the Arms

● **Triceps**: The triceps are located on the backside of the upper arm. The triceps make up two-thirds of the upper arm. Their primary function is to extend (straighten) the upper arm when the elbow joint is isolated. They assist the pectorals and deltoids when performing any pressing movement. Primary exercises for the triceps are the french curl and triceps extension.

● **Biceps**: The biceps compose one-third of your upper arm. Their primary function is to flex the upper arm. Your biceps assist the latissimus dorsi any time a pulling movement is performed. A primary exercise for the biceps would be any form of a biceps curl.

● **Forearm Flexors**: The forearm flexors are located on the bottom side of the forearm (when the palms are facing the floor). Their primary function during exercise is to grip and to flex the wrist. They are the muscles used to grip. Some of the activities involving the use of grip strength are chinups, negotiating a horizontal ladder, climbing a rope, squeezing a tennis racquet, etc. Wrist flexion can be observed in activities similar to throwing, or shooting a basketball. A primary exercise for the forearm flexors is the wrist curl.

Muscles of the Neck

There is an abundance of individual muscles composing the muscle groups of the neck. To simplify the identification of the neck muscles and their function, they are categorized as flexors, extensors, and lateral flexors.

● **Flexors**: The function of the flexors is to bend the head forward. These muscles are primarily located on the front side of your neck. The neck curl exercise is an exercise specific to the neck flexors. The greatest percentage of severe neck injuries occurs when the neck is hyperflexed.

● **Extensors**: The function of the extensors is to bend your head backward. These muscles are primarily located on the back side of the head. The neck extension exercise is a primary exercise for the neck extensors.

● **Lateral Flexors**: The primary function of the lateral flexors is to bend your head sideward. These muscles are located on both sides of the neck. The lateral flexion exercise is a primary exercise for the lateral flexors.

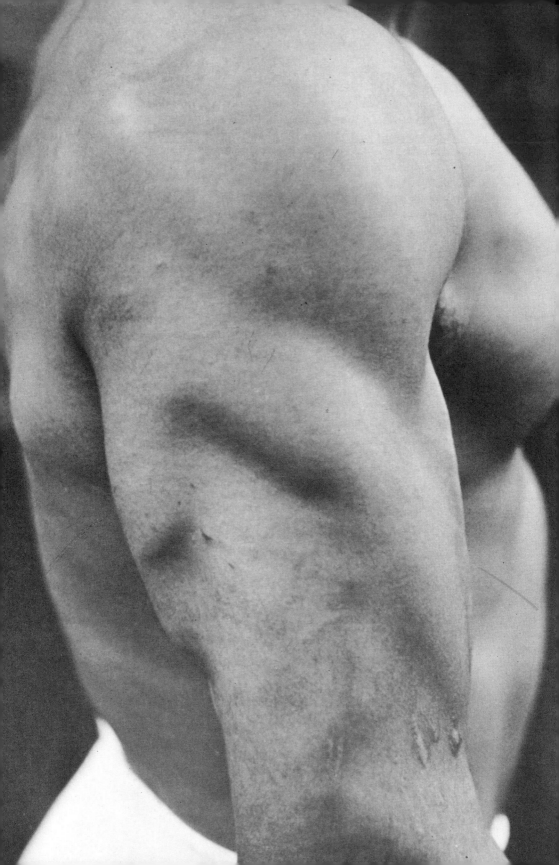

3

MUSCLES: STRUCTURE, FUNCTION, AND CONTROL

by
Michael D. Wolf, Ph.D.

Fast twitch. Slow twitch. Red muscle. White muscle. Chances are you've run into one or more of these terms in your travels, and not having a degree in muscle biochemistry, wondered what they meant to you as a coach, trainer, or athlete. The following is an overview of the structure, function, and control of human muscle, always keeping in mind that such knowledge is going to be applied to training and sport.

Q. HOW DOES MUSCLE CONTRACT?

A. Human muscle is, somewhat surprisingly to the non-scientist, over 70% water. Approximately 22% of muscle tissue is protein. Of this latter percentage, the majority is accounted for by millions of strands of a thin filament protein called **actin** and a thick filament protein called **myosin.** Given the presence of calcium, magnesium, and two other proteins called **troponin** and **tropomyosin,** these two filament proteins can contract and move your limbs with great force and great velocity.

The fuel for muscular contraction is a chemical compound called **adenosine triphosphate**, or ATP. When one of the three phosphates is broken off ATP to form ADP, or **adenosine diphosphate**, energy is released into the muscular environment (Figure 1). When actin binds to myosin in the presence of calcium, the energy released from ATP breakdown is used to **pull the actin filaments along the myosin filaments.** More specifically, a bridge forms between actin and myosin. Energy from ATP breakdown is used to shorten the **actomyosin cross-bridge**, which shortens the muscle.

27

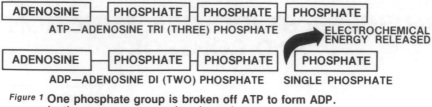

ATP—ADENOSINE TRI (THREE) PHOSPHATE

ADP—ADENOSINE DI (TWO) PHOSPHATE   SINGLE PHOSPHATE

Figure 1 **One phosphate group is broken off ATP to form ADP.
In the process, energy is released.**

Figure 2 shows a simplified unit of muscle called a **sarcomere**. One long strand of many thousands of sarcomeres is called a **myofibril** (Figure 3). Many myofibrils bundled together form one **muscle fiber**. Given the proper input from the nervous system, innervated (switched-on) sarcomeres will contract, and the muscle as a whole will shorten (Figure 4). The process was detailed and named the "Sliding Filament Theory" more than 20 years ago by noted British physiologist H.E. Huxley. Huxley has been internationally honored for his since-proven theory, and is presently Deputy Director of the Molecular Biology Laboratory at Cambridge University in England.

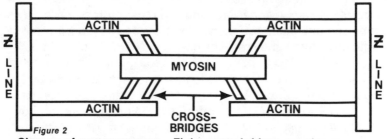

Figure 2

**Closeup of one sarcomere. Eight cross-bridges are shown
extending from myosin to actin. Given energy from ATP breakdown,
these cross-bridges attach to the actin filaments, shorten and
telescope the entire Z-line filament units over the myosin filament.**

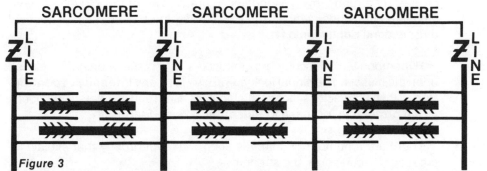

Figure 3
A schematic diagram of three sarcomeres from one myofilament.
Many thousands of sarcomeres form just one myofilament.
Refer to figure 2 for explanation.

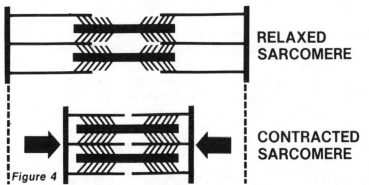

RELAXED
SARCOMERE

CONTRACTED
SARCOMERE

Figure 4
When cross-bridges pull Z-lines together, sarcomere length
decreases, but neither actin nor myosin filaments shorten.

Q. HOW DOES MUSCLE GROW?

A. The technical term for muscular growth is **hypertrophy**. Its inverse, called **atrophy**, refers to the breakdown of muscle tissue from disuse. The process of atrophy involves metabolic breakdown of muscle into its constituent compounds, which are removed via the bloodstream. Atrophied muscle **does not** turn into fat.

Hypertrophy, or muscular growth, occurs as a result of demands placed upon the muscle. The signal for hypertrophy is clearly **intensity of contraction**. When a muscle is faced with high intensity requirements, it responds with a **protective increase in muscular size and strength**.

There are a number of changes seen with hypertrophy that explain increased muscular size and strength:
- The actin and particularly the myosin protein filaments increase in size.
- The number of myofibrils (lengths of actin/myosin units, or "sarcomeres") increases.
- The number of blood capillaries within the fiber may increase.
- The amount and strength of connective tissue within the muscle may increase.
- The number of muscle fibers (which consist of many myofibrils) may increase.

There is heavy scientific debate over the occurrence of this last phenomenon, which is called **hyperplasia.** While a small number of studies on rats and cats have shown hyperplasia, or **fiber splitting** with increased muscular size, most researchers have not been able to demonstrate it. As of 1981, there is no evidence that the number of muscle fibers increases in humans when muscular size and strength are increased through weight training.

Q. ARE THERE DIFFERENT TYPES OF MUSCLE?

A. In the middle 1970's there was some debate over just how many types of muscle could be found in humans. International consensus has since firmly established a four-category classification of human muscle. The only confusion that exists at present is in the naming of the categories. There is no disagreement in international circles over the fact that four distinct types of muscle fiber exist in man, however. Table 1 presents the three major classification schemes for the four types of human muscle fiber.

The four fiber types differ on a great number of characteristics. The three most important are force of contraction, speed of contraction, and endurance.

Table 1

THREE CLASSIFICATION SCHEMES

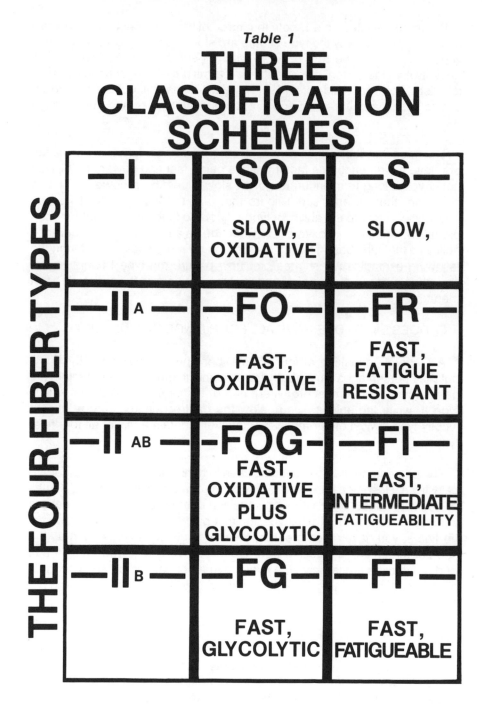

THE FOUR FIBER TYPES		
—I—	—SO— SLOW, OXIDATIVE	—S— SLOW,
—IIA—	—FO— FAST, OXIDATIVE	—FR— FAST, FATIGUE RESISTANT
—II AB—	—FOG— FAST, OXIDATIVE PLUS GLYCOLYTIC	—FI— FAST, INTERMEDIATE FATIGUEABILITY
—IIB—	—FG— FAST, GLYCOLYTIC	—FF— FAST, FATIGUEABLE

Referring back to Table 1, note that three of the four fiber types are characterized as fast. Only the type I fibers are slow in contraction speed. They were once called the red, or slow-twitch fibers, but the "red-white" and "slow-twitch, fast twitch" classification systems are no longer used by physiologists. The word "oxidative" (Table 1) refers to the ability of the muscle tissue to use oxygen for long periods of time to synthesize and make use of ATP.

The three fast fibers differ from each other most in endurance. The IIa fibers have a high endurnce factor despite being fast and powerful. They do not have the long-term endurance of the slow, type I fibers, however. The IIb fibers are the powerful sprint fibers that fatigue most quickly. The term "glycolytic" refers to the ability of type II fibers to function well, but for short periods of time, without oxygen. Between the IIa and IIb fibers in endurance ability lie the IIab fibers. Though the issue is far more complicated than the following examples will suggest, for now picture the type I fibers as the marathon runner's "best friend" and the type IIb fibers as the sprinter's "best friend."

Q. DOES EVERYONE HAVE ALL FOUR KINDS OF MUSCLE?

A. Generally speaking, all four muscle fiber types can be seen in the body, but their percentages vary greatly from muscle to muscle. For example, the gastrocnemius (the most prominent part of the calf) can be almost wholly type II, while the soleus, lying below the gastrocnemius, can be almost wholly type I. Most of our muscles, however, contain a mix of all four fiber types.

The percentage of each fiber type seen in a muscle appears to be genetically fixed. Research has shown fairly conclusively that training has a small or negligible effect on the fiber composition of muscle. What that means is this: if you were born with deltoids and triceps that are largely composed of IIb fibers, you have much greater potential in athletic events such as the shotput than if those muscles were type I. Conversely, if your hamstrings and quadriceps are largely type I you have an enhanced potential for success at distance running. To a great extent, elite athletes are born and not made.

Q. HOW DOES THE BRAIN CALL UPON AND USE MUSCLE?

A. It was once thought that the thin, gray **motor cortex**, sitting on top of the brain, was in complete control of movement. Plans were made, commands issued downward, and the muscle snapped into action. It is now known that the motor cortex is the **last** brain structure to act before movement, rather than the **first**. Plans appear to be made in the **frontal cortex**, movements initiated and coordinated in the **basal ganglia** and **cerebellum** then relayed through the thalamus, and final commands directed from **motor cortex** downward into the **spinal cord.** It is also known that there are a number of spinal pathways that can carry commands from brain centers **other than the motor cortex** directly to the muscle (Figure 5).

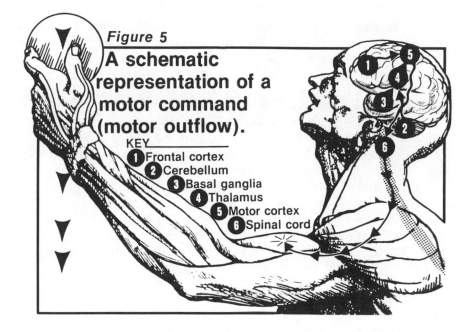

Figure 5

A schematic representation of a motor command (motor outflow).

KEY
1. Frontal cortex
2. Cerebellum
3. Basal ganglia
4. Thalamus
5. Motor cortex
6. Spinal cord

When a message from any of the brain centers, called **supraspinal** (above the spine) **centers**, reaches the spinal cord, it is transmitted to the muscle via the **motorneuron**. These structures are simply nerves that carry motor commands. The number of muscle fibers that one motorneuron can control varies from as little as one to as many as several hundred. One motorneuron, and **all** the muscle fibers it controls, is called a **motor unit**. When a motorneuron turns on its muscle fibers, they must contract fully in one burst. The principle that an individual muscle fiber is either completely "on" or completely "off" is called the **all-or-none law.**

The natural question that the all-or-none law raises is: "How can we get different forces of contraction, or **graded contraction**, if muscle fibers are either on or off?" The answer is that the brain only calls on the number and types of muscle fibers that it needs. When the need for more force arises, the brain has a number of options. One of these is to simply ask or **recruit** more all-or-none fibers. The other is to stimulate the fibers it **has already called on**, or **recruited**, more rapidly. There is a sizeable debate going on concerning how much the brain relies on "more fibers" versus "faster stimulation" when more force is needed.

To summarize thus far, the brain estimates the number and type of fibers it needs for a task, then recruits them in an all-or-none fashion. If these fibers are not enough, the brain will do one of several things:

- Stimulate the already-on fibers more rapidly (frequency)
- Ask for more of the same fibers to join in (recruitment)
- Ask for fibers of a **more powerful** type to join in (recruitment)

Hidden in this last sentence is perhaps the most important point in this whole discussion. There is a wealth of evidence that in nearly all human endeavors the brain follows the **size principle of recruitment**. This principle states that recruitment order is based upon increasing size of motorneurons. Most simply, small motorneurons are called upon first, and the largest motorneurons are recruited last. Since muscle fiber size correlates closely with the size order of motorneurons, the type I fibers (the smallest) are recruited first, and the type IIb (the largest) are recruited last.

Nearly all evidence suggests that in humans it is the **intensity or force requirements** that determine which and how many muscle fibers will be used. There is no evidence that the speed of contraction determines fiber recruitment. In other words, the brain recruits muscle based on how much force the muscle must create, and not on how fast it must contract. The simple explanation for this is that so-called "slow-twitch" or type I fibers are fully capable of moving the limbs at extreme velocities (greater than 1000 degrees per second) **if the force requirements are low**. Training rapidly but with low intensity **cannot** prepare the muscle for high intensity athletic performance.

For low intensity muscular work, the small type I fibers (the smallest of the four types) will suffice. Once the type I fibers become insufficient for the task, the brain will recruit the next **larger** fiber types or the IIa or IIab fibers. When even the I, IIa, and IIab fibers cannot meet the force requirements the brain will, **as a last resort**, recruit the largest type IIb fibers. All **four** fiber types are working when IIb fibers are recruited. Athletic performance requiring movements of power and speed utilize all four fiber types but are most dependent on the IIb fibers. There is **no** firm evidence in humans that **any movement**, at **any speed,** can cause the brain to **preferentially recruit IIb [formerly "fast-twitch"] fibers**. Such preferential recruitment, the bypassing of I, IIa, and IIab fibers, has been shown in extremely rapid, low force movements in cats, but no researcher has been able to demonstrate it in humans.

Q. WHY THEN DO MANY COACHES AND EQUIPMENT MANUFACTURERS ADVOCATE HIGH SPEED TRAINING?

A. Such training advice can be blamed on a lack of knowledge of basic neuromuscular physiology and a great deal of poorly-conducted research. Most laymen, and unfortunately many exercise researchers, assume that slow-twitch (type I) fibers are only responsible for slow movements. As noted above, the type I fibers may move a limb at extreme speeds **if the load is light**. Once loading assumes the proportions of a 200 pound offensive lineman, type IIa and IIb fibers must also be recruited. Neglect of these neurophysiological principles has been based on several widely-published studies, but none as much as the work by Moffroid and Whipple (1970) in the Journal of The American Physical Therapy Association.

The authors trained one experimental group on isokinetic knee extension at a high intensity and low speed (36 degrees per second). A second experimental group was trained at what the authors **called** a fast speed. Since human limbs may exceed one thousand degrees per second in angular velocity, it is clear that this second group, training at 108 degrees per second, was not training at a high speed. Nevertheless, this latter speed has been accepted by the community as "fast." A third group was tested before and after the six week training period, but was not trained. After the six weeks, the three groups were tested at zero degrees per second (isometrically) and at six speeds from 18 to 108 degrees per second.

Moffroid and Whipple conducted that training at a "fast" speed led to strength gains at all speeds tested while the "slow" group only gained in strength at slow speeds. **This conclusion has been cited literally hundreds of times since 1970 as evidence that training should occur at high speed and low intensity.** The data from Moffroid and Whipple (1970) are presented here exactly as they appeared in print (Table 2), and both of the original peak torque curves (which had appeared separately) are plotted for comparison on one graph (Figure 6).

35

Table 2

Mean Increases of Peak Torque for Quadriceps

Velocity	Group I (Newton Meters) SLOW	Group II (Newton Meters) FAST	Group III (Newton Meters) CONTROL
0 rpm	28.6	21.8	14.1
3 rpm	35.4	16.8	3.9
6 rpm	47.1	24.8	8.3
9 rpm	14.5	14.5	8.4
12 rpm	14.1	17.5	6.9
15 rpm	10.8	12.3	4.8
18 rpm	8.4	15.6	2.0

from: M. MOFFROID & R WHIPPLE. SPECIFICITY OF SPEED AND EXERCISE. JOURNAL OF THE AMERICAN PHYSICAL THERAPY ASSOCIATION Volume 50 : 1699, 1970.

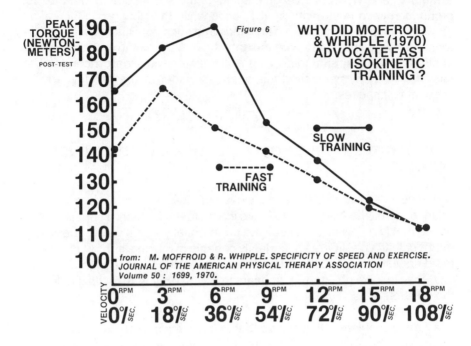

PEAK TORQUE (NEWTON-METERS) POST-TEST

Figure 6

WHY DID MOFFROID & WHIPPLE (1970) ADVOCATE FAST ISOKINETIC TRAINING ?

SLOW TRAINING

FAST TRAINING

from: *M. MOFFROID & R. WHIPPLE. SPECIFICITY OF SPEED AND EXERCISE. JOURNAL OF THE AMERICAN PHYSICAL THERAPY ASSOCIATION Volume 50 : 1699, 1970.*

VELOCITY

The data absolutely do not support the authors' conclusions. If for no other reason, the conclusions are valueless because the authors violated a basic principle of statistical analysis: when pre-tests indicated that one group had higher mean peak torques at all speeds, analysis of **post-test** data should have employed a technique known as "analysis of covariance." This tool **statistically equates** the two groups on **pre-test** data so that **post-test** results can be compared fairly. Given the initial differences found by Moffroid and Whipple, their use of analysis of variance, and not **co**variance, prevents consideration of any of their conclusions.

Despite this failure, the results can be reinspected. A close analysis of the data reveals that the **only statistically significant differences** between groups were at two lower speeds, where the slow group showed nearly **twice** the gains of the fast group (Table 2). In the case where fast outgained slow, the differences were not only of much smaller magnitude, but **were not statistically significant**. In layman's terms, failure to reach significance means only one thing: the differences **cannot be attributed to training method**.

Moffroid and Whipple, even in the light of the above, stated that the fast group increased in strength at all speeds while the slow group increased only at slow speeds. It should be obvious that such conclusions were incorrect and totally unsupported by the data. In fact, according to the principles of statistics and experimental design, all their analyses were incorrect. It is sad that so many have cited this study as evidence that training should occur at fast speeds.

Q. WHAT THEN IS THE MOST EFFECTIVE WAY TO STRENGTHEN MUSCLE?

A. There is solid evidence that slow, high intensity training causes the brain to recruit the I, IIa, and IIb fibers in an orderly fashion. There is no evidence that fast, low intensity training preferentially works the IIb fibers. Remember that type I fibers are perfectly capable of moving limbs at extremely rapid speeds (over 1000 degrees per second) if the force requirements are low. Training at high intensity appears to be the **only way** to maximally use the IIb fibers.

A further problem with high speed training is that the only way to move a heavy load rapidly is to "explode" into it. Two very definite things occur with explosive movement, and both of them are unacceptable and potentially destructive.

In terms of safety, the forces created in such a movement can easily exceed the structural integrity of muscle, connective and bone tissue. Explosive training is, sooner or later, a sure ticket to the orthopedic surgeon's office.

Furthermore, when a barbell or load is moved explosively, the weight is given sufficient momentum to work under its own power. Such movement is called **ballistic**. Note on the oscilloscope tracing in Figure 7 that the load on the muscles in an explosive, 60 pound barbell military press is **below** 60 pounds for almost half the movement! Quite obviously, if the load on the muscle significantly decreases below 60 pounds, the muscle is **not being trained**. Given the inherent dangers and the ineffective loading of the musculature, one wonders why any athlete would be coached to train explosively.

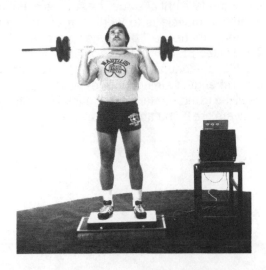

Figure 7. A force plate is a measuring device that is used to measure changes in force. Pictured above is a subject standing on a force plate that is connected to an oscilloscope. As the subject performs an overhead press, the forces are recorded. If the movement is performed in a smooth, steady manner, the signal on the screen will travel across the scope in a relatively straight line fashion. If the barbell is pressed in a fast, explosive style, the signal will move wildly up and down the scope, thereby accurately indicating the changing levels of force imposed upon the subject.

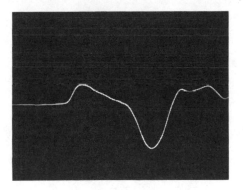

An actual tracing of the changing forces involved in rapid exercise is shown in this photo. Notice the peaks and drops in the tracing. A 60-pound barbell—if suddenly jerked or thrown—can exert a force of several hundred pounds, or can exert a force that literally measures below zero! Such rapid exercise is not only unproductive as far as strength training is concerned, but is also very dangerous to the joints, muscles, and connective tissues.

In conclusion, the great weight of evidence suggests that the most effective way to train human muscle is to work it at great intensity and slow speed. Research and experience from major projects at Colorado State University and The United States Military Academy at West Point, and ongoing work at Nautilus headquarters in Lake Helen, Florida, support the concept that optimal strength training requires as little as one set of eight to twelve repetitions taken to momentary muscular failure. Many questions remain, but their answers are being actively pursued.

4

STRENGTH TRAINING MISCONCEPTIONS

by
Bill Dervrich
University of Iowa

If only Milo the Greek knew of the misconceptions and idiosyncrasies that would evolve from the time he started lifting that baby bull nearly two thousand years ago, he would have stopped after his first lift. However, since that time of the first lift by Milo, research in strength training has produced new techniques and theories to be used in conditioning and training of athletes. Yet an endless list of myths, superstitions, and questionable practices continue to be incorporated into many strength training programs.

If you want to improve your level of muscular fitness as much as possible, you must first separate fact from intuition. An effective strength training program must be based on scientific principles, not intuitive misconceptions and misfounded practices. This chapter examines a few of the well known misconceptions regarding strength training.

EFFECTS OF STRENGTH TRAINING ON WOMEN

It is a common misconception among women that if they participate in a strength training program the end results will be massive bulging muscles. There are, however, many anatomical differences between men and women that will affect an individual's ability to develop muscle strength and size. The most significant difference between the females and males is the level of testosterone. Testosterone is a hormone which affects the development of the muscle. The higher level of testosterone, the greater the potential for increasing both the muscle's size and strength. The average male possesses a much higher level of testosterone than does the average female. Due to the fact that women possess lower levels of testosterone in the blood, their potential for increasing the muscle size and strength is much lower than that of males.

One study conducted on women athletes, for example, indicated that women can increase their muscular strength by forty-four percent with no adverse affects on the size of the muscle. It can then be stated that the development of the muscle's size and strength will be directly proportionate to the muscle's growth potential. Due to her certain genetic differences, a woman does not possess the same muscular growth potential as a man.

Another physiological variable preventing or minimizing the existence of bulging muscles in women is the higher percentage of fat levels in the body. With the female possessing a higher level of fat per pound of bodyweight, the size potential of the muscles is limited.

Society's suppression of females physically has undoubtedly prevented many women from developing to their maximum physical potential. For that reason alone, women have more to gain from a properly organized strength training program than do men. There is nothing unfeminine about a woman who cares enough about her body to take care of it. Women have both a right and an obligation to be muscularly fit.

SPEED OF MOVEMENT

Many coaches and athletes believe that an increase in the size and strength of a muscle will result in slower movements when performing a particular athletic skill. Actually, just the opposite takes place. The speed at which you can perform a particular movement will be enhanced tremendously by increasing your strength levels. The speed of a body movement is dependent on two factors: the strength of the muscles that are actually involved when performing a specific skill and your capacity to recruit muscle fibers while performing the movement (neurological efficiency).

It is fallacious to assume that a muscle will "slow down" by increasing its strength and size. The correlation between the speed of a muscle movement and the strength level of the muscle are positively related. Therefore, to increase the speed of a muscle movement, increase the strength levels of the muscles needed to perform that particular movement.

MARATHON WORKOUTS

The length of each strength training workout that an individual undertakes in the weight room is a constant source of disagreement among lifters. It has long been the American way that the more I do, the better I will become. Many coaches and athletes, for example, strongly believe that a two to three hour workout is necessary to obtain maximum gains in strength. While this may be true for many activities, it cannot be said for strength training. To dispel this myth, you should observe what occurs during the typical two hour strength training workout. You will obviously see that a good portion of the workout is spent talking, changing weights, and allowing too much time between actual lifts.

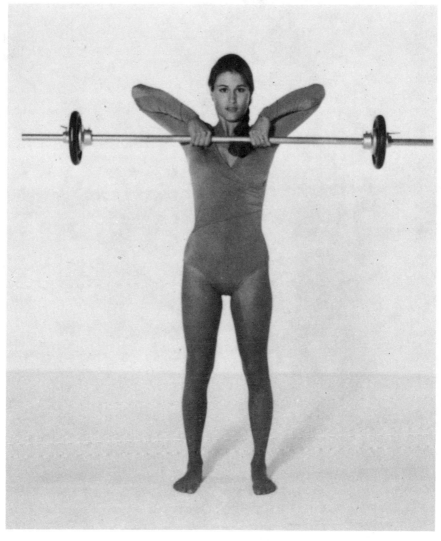

Women have more to gain from a properly organized strength program than do men.

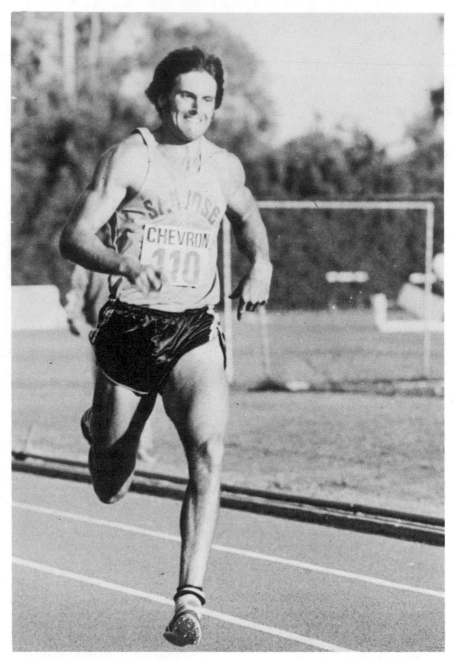

It is fallacious to assume that a muscle will "slow down" by increasing its strength and size.

In 1975, a study was conducted at the United States Military Academy to examine the consequences of a short duration, high intensity strength training program. The results from the study showed that maximum strength gains can be produced by performing only three workouts per week with each workout consuming less than twenty minutes. The research also refuted the erroneous belief that an effective strength training program must be too time consuming—a main reason why some athletic programs refuse to avoid including time for strength training. They feel that they don't have the time. But they do. They must.

It is imperative to remember that all work being performed in the weight room should focus on quality, not quantity. A properly organized and well executed strength training program will increase new levels of strength while consuming a small amount of time.

MUSCLE BOUND

One misconception that individuals constantly argue over is the definition of a muscle bound athlete. Muscle bound is a term used to describe a muscular person who does not have adequate flexibility or movement. The first usage of this term was during the 19th Century and related to the strong men of the traveling circuses. Such individuals whose movements were generally slow and awkward were restricted by their massiveness. However, most of the massiveness of these individuals was in the form of fat. On one hand, these individuals were able to increase their bodyweight by fifty to a hundred pounds with most of that additional weight in the form of fat. On the other hand, that dead weight (fat) greatly reduced their levels of agility, mobility, coordination, and flexibility. Since these individuals were very strong, the people of this era drew a close relation between massiveness and lack of movement.

Unfortunately, many individuals today continue to believe that increase in the size of the muscle will produce symptoms associated with muscle boundness. Contradictory to this belief is the latest research that supports the theory that a well organized strength training program can enhance both size and strength without adversely affecting the individual's coordination, agility, mobility, and flexibility.

PROTEIN SUPPLEMENTS

Many individuals believe that consuming large quantities of protein will give them an edge in developing massive muscles and will shorten the amount of time required to build such muscles.

Some individuals feel that since a muscle is composed of a substantial amount of protein, the consumption of large amounts of protein will facilitate the development of a muscle rapidly in both size and strength. However, it is physiologically impossible for the body to perform such a function. What research has found is that the muscles are seventy percent water, twenty-two percent protein, and seven percent lipids. Only after a muscle is drained of water and fluids will protein remain. But many individuals fail to study all the data. Moreover, they want to believe that muscles are made of protein because it justifies centuries of meat eating. Surveys show that many individuals consume four to five times their protein requirements each day. There is absolutely no performance benefit from consuming large amounts of protein.

Research has also shown that a balanced diet provides more protein than any individual, including athletes, needs. Food items that supply the highest quality of proteins come from beef, pork, fish, chicken, eggs, and dairy products. Additional protein that is not absorbed by the body is eliminated through the excretory system.

Furthermore, a potential danger exists to people who consume large amounts of protein. Recent studies suggest that excessive amounts of protein may be harmful to a person's kidneys and liver.

Although a protein supplement may provide a boost mentally from a physiological standpoint, it is both unsound and a waste of money.

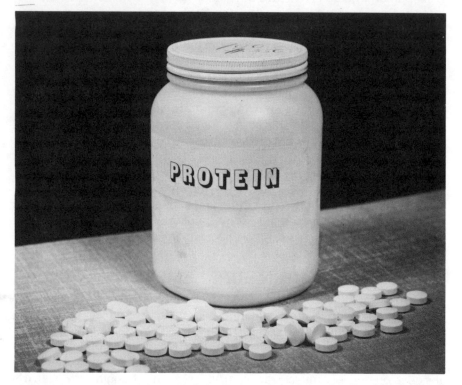

Ingesting protein supplements is both an unsound practice (healthwise) and a waste of money.

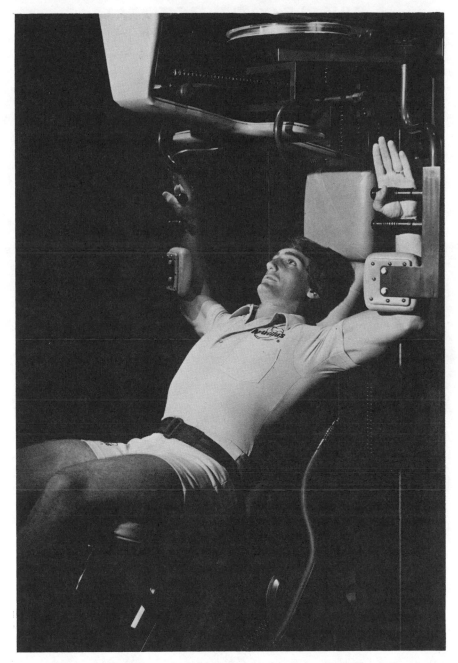

Proper strength training not only does not decrease flexibility, it increases flexibility.

MUSCLE CONVERTS TO FAT

It is a common misconception among coaches and athletes, in particular, that muscle, when no longer stimulated through exercise, will transform to fat.

If you were to chemically analyze fat and muscle, you would discover that muscle and fat both contain varying amounts of water, protein, and lipid substances. However, when muscle is exercised, it will contract and produce a movement, whereas fat will not contract and is usually stored in the body as a source of fuel. It is physiologically and chemically impossible to convert muscle to fat and vice-versa.

A simple explanation of what takes place can be illustrated by observing the ex-athlete's pattern of exercise and caloric intake. When an athlete stops exercising his/her muscles, the muscles will begin to atrophy. At the same time, that athlete will continue to consume the same level of calories. With the athlete consuming more calories than are needed to maintain his/her energy demands, the excess is then stored in the body as additional fat. If an athlete becomes obese after terminating a strength training program, it is due to caloric imbalance (eating more than expending) and not muscle transforming to fat.

Some individuals believe that their bodyweight should maintain a constant level upon the termination of a strength training program. Unfortunately, these individuals fail to understand that if they lose ten pounds of muscle mass through muscle atrophy and their body weight remains the same, then the weight loss that is attributed to muscle atrophy has been replaced by deposits of additional fat.

Upon the completion of any strength training program, the development of new eating habits, commensurate with a new life style, must be cultivated to maintain proper body fat levels.

Darden, Ellington, *Nutrition and Athletic Performance.* Pasadena: The Athletic Press, 1976.

Peterson, James A. "Total Conditioning: A Case Study," *Athletic Journal*, 56:40-55, September, 1975.

5

GENETIC FACTORS AFFECTING STRENGTH DEVELOPMENT

by
Daniel P. Riley
Washington Redskins

Obviously, all individuals are not made from the same physical mold. Therefore, all individuals are not capable of running at the same speed, jumping the same height, lifting the same amount of weight, and so on. Your genetic potential for physical performance is determined at birth. Other factors also affect your potential for success. The environment, for example, in which you exist may eliminate or reduce the possibility of your ever engaging in any activity in which you possess the potential for greatness. You, for example, may possess all of the physical attributes and characteristics needed to become a championship golfer. However, if you live in an area where there is no golf course, your potential for greatness will probably never be developed due to factors beyond your control.

As you approach the higher levels of athletic competition, a process of natural selection begins to evolve. The average or below average athlete is frequently "weeded out" due to a deficiency in genetic makeup. Many athletes obtain a moderate degree of success in sports but very few possess the physical attributes needed to obtain the highest levels of performance.

Remember that the function of an activity will dictate the physical attributes which are essential to success in that endeavor. It is not by chance that the tall athlete finds success in basketball, or that the big and powerful athlete excels in football. The nature of these activities demands a unique combination of physical and mental attributes which allow the athlete to excel.

The noted exercise physiologist, Karpovich, perhaps put it best when he stated, "Men who look alike may have such differences in physiological functions that some become champion athletes while others remain ordinary mortals. The importance of individual differences and aptitudes is well recognized. No coach in his right mind would attempt to make a champion out of just anybody. No amount of training will transform a thick set, round-bellied individual into a track champion. It is like trying to make a greyhound out of a Saint Bernard. A coach must select promising material before attempting to train it."

One of the purposes of this chapter is to make the reader aware of some of the more obvious anatomical attributes that are needed to significantly increase muscle mass and strength. Remember that your potential for increasing muscle strength and size was determined at birth by your genetic makeup. If you possess all of these attributes in the proper combination, you have a greater potential for increasing muscle mass and strength than the person who doesn't possess this same combination of physiological and biochemical advantages. Among the attributes that affect your potential to develop strength are bodytype, length of the lever, and muscle belly length.

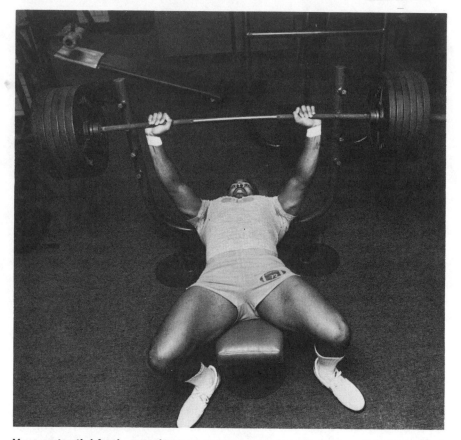

Your potential for increasing your muscle mass and size was determined at birth by your genetic make-up.

BODYTYPE

A person's bodytype (also known as somatype) describes a distinct type of body structure. Essentially, it refers to the size of the bones, the bone structure of the body, and the percentage of muscle and fat covering the bones of the body.

Bodytypes can be categorized into three broad and very general groups: ectomorphs, mesomorphs, and endomorphs. These three basic bodytypes allow an individual to be identified by bodytype if he/she possesses certain characteristics. This identification process is complicated by the fact that most people possess characteristics from more than one category of bodytype.

The three primary bodytypes have definitive attributes.

● **Ectomorph:** The ectomorph possesses predominant characteristics of linearity, fragility, small bones, thin muscles and little fat. Those individuals possessing qualities of the ectomorph have little potential for gaining high levels of muscle strength and mass. The cross country runner is an example of a person possessing some of the ectomorphic qualities.

● **Mesomorph:** The mesomorph is characterized by a square body with hard, rugged, and prominent musculation with little fat. The mesomorph's bones are large and covered with thick muscle. Mesomorphs have the greatest potential for gaining muscle mass and strength. Wrestlers, gymnasts and football linemen are examples of individuals who possess a high level of the mesomorphic characteristics. The activities of the mesomorph demand a need for speed, power, and strength with little need for fat.

● **Endomorph:** The pure endomorph is characterized by roundness and softness of the body. A very high percentage of fat is present. The true endomorph exhibits very little potential for anything except inactivity and consuming large quantities of food.

LENGTH OF THE LEVER (BONE)

Your body is a system of levers with the bones of the body serving as the levers. You should take into consideration the length of your levers when trying to determine why you may or may not be stronger than other people.

Because your arms or legs are used in most exercises, their length will have a significant effect on your ability to overcome a resistance when performing most exercises. The formula for work (work = force × distance) can give you insight to the mechanics of the problem. An individual with long arms will have to perform more work while raising a weight than would a person with shorter arms raising that same weight. The individual with the longer arms would be moving the resistance a greater distance (performing more work) than would the person with shorter arms. When determining who could lift more weight, you should assume (all other things being equal) that if you have short arms, you would have a mechanical advantage over the person with longer arms. It is not unreasonable to conclude then that a weak long-levered athlete is therefore at a distinct disadvantage, for he/she can employ his/her levers against only very light resistances.

INSERTION POINT OF THE MUSCLE

For a muscle to produce movement it must be connected to two bones. One of the two bones is often more moveable than the other. For example, Figure 5-1 illustrates how one end of the biceps attaches to the upper arm (at the shoulder) and the other end to the forearm. When the muscle contracts, the more moveable bone (the lower arm) is moved toward the less moveable one (the upper arm). The point of attachment to the less moveable bone is called the origin of the muscle and the point of attachment to the more moveable bone is called the insertion.

In the human body, the point of origin is generally in the same place on a bone. The point of origin therefore will not affect the mechanical advantage of muscle and bone involved. However, the point of insertion varies with each individual. The farther away from the joint that the muscle inserts, the better the mechanical advantage will be (Figures 5-2 to 5-4).

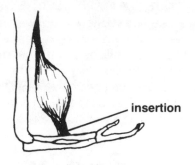

Figure 5-1
The biceps attaches to the arm.

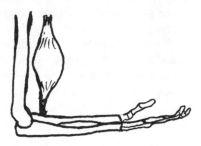

Figure 5-2
Average mechanical advantage.

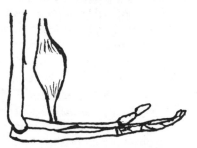

Figure 5-3
Better mechanical advantage.

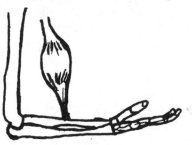

Figure 5-4
Best mechanical advantage.

Dyson, the noted exercise physiologist, confirmed that some individuals are indeed born with an advantage: "Some athletes, fortunately endowed, possess muscular insertions that are further from their joints than the average person; and this, if true of one of their bone levers, appears to apply to them all! Only a very small difference is necessary to give considerable mechanical advantage."

The two genetic factors previously mentioned (the length of the lever and the point of insertion of the muscle) together, could be the difference between whether or not you're an average performer or a champion.

NEUROMUSCULAR EFFICIENCY

Neuromuscular efficiency refers to your ability to recruit muscle fibers through the signals transmitted by the central nervous system. Some individuals have a very efficient neuromuscular system which allows them to recruit a higher percentage of muscle fibers when performing an exercise or activity. This conscious recruitment of muscle fibers may prove to be the critical genetic factor accounting for the difference between two athletes who appear to be blessed with the same mechanical and physiological advantages.

For example, hypothetically, you can observe two athletes who are identical twins. The length of their levers and points of insertion are identical. The size of the muscles and everything about the two individuals may appear to be identical. The only differences between the two athletes is their level of neuromuscular efficiency.

In theory, however, if twin #1 has a neuromuscular system that is 10% more efficient than twin #2, this neurological difference will provide twin #1 with a greater potential for recruiting muscle fibers when performing a specific exercise or activity. While exerting an all out physical effort, twin #1 will have the greater potential for achieving a higher level of success than twin #2.

QUALITY AND LENGTH

Two other factors that probably play a very important role in your ability to gain strength and muscle mass are the percentage of red and white muscle fibers and the length of the belly of a muscle. For discussion purposes, assume that you have primarily two different types or qualities of muscle fibers in your body. These different fiber types are referred to as red muscle fibers (slow twitch) and white muscle fibers (fast twitch). White muscle fiber primarily contributes to activities which involve explosive power, short bursts of speed, anaerobic strength and endurance. It appears that the white muscle fibers, when trained, possess a greater potential for increasing muscle strength and mass. If true, the individual who is blessed with a high percentage of white muscle fibers should have a greater potential for increasing power, muscle strength and size.

Red muscle fiber primarily contributes to activities involving the continuous contraction of a muscle over an extended period of time. Red muscle fiber has a greater affinity for myoglobin which allows it to utilize oxygen with a greater efficiency than a white muscle fiber. Therefore, aerobic activities place the greatest demand on red fibers, while anaerobic exercises primarily utilize white muscle fibers.

If this is the case, it appears that the highly successful distance runner, for example, would possess a higher percentage of red muscle fiber than of white muscle fiber. A distance runner, therefore, possesses limited potential for developing a high level of strength and muscle mass.

On the other hand, a successful football player would probably possess a very high percentage of white muscle fiber and a low percentage of red muscle fiber. Consequently, his potential for increasing muscle mass and strength is very high while his potential for becoming a successful distance runner is very low.

To better understand this phenomenon look at the muscle fibers of a common barnyard turkey. While observing the daily activities of the turkey, you can see it spending an enormous amount of time walking around the barnyard using the muscles of the legs (drumsticks) continuously. Therefore, the quality of the muscle fibers used to provide this constant movement must be capable of contracting over an extended period of time or that of the red muscle fiber. When eating a turkey leg, note that the meat is dark in color. The red muscle fiber theory is supported.

While observing this same turkey, note that it very seldom ventures into the air to fly. One of the reasons that the turkey does not possess the potential for flying long distances may be because the muscles used to fly (chest muscles) do not possess the quality of muscle fibers needed for endurance on extended flight. The turkey can make a few strong, violent contractions with the wings but cannot continue these contractions with the wings for any length of time. The breast meat of the turkey is white (muscle fiber).

The percentage of white and red muscle fibers will vary with each muscle fiber. The person who possesses the proper combination of all of the previously mentioned genetic factors, in addition to a higher percentage of white muscle fibers, will probably have the greatest potential for increasing muscle mass and strength.

MUSCLE BELLY LENGTH

If your tendon were severed from the muscle, the muscle belly would remain (Figure 5-5). The cross-sectional area of the individual muscle fiber can be significantly increased but its length is fixed. Therefore, a muscle is limited to what extent it can develop (size-wise) by the length of its belly.

Consequently, (with all other things remaining equal), if you are blessed with muscles with a long belly, you have a greater potential for increasing muscle mass and strength than someone with shorter muscle bellies. This phenomenon certainly applies to every muscle group in your body.

Figure 5-6 illustrates how the length of a muscle can affect its ability to develop. Obviously one calf muscle possesses a much longer muscle belly than the other. The calf muscle with the longer muscle belly (on the right) should possess the greatest potential for increasing muscle mass and strength.

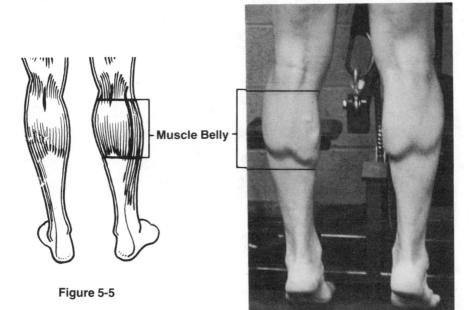

Figure 5-5

Figure 5-6

CONCLUSION

Too often, the athlete, weightlifter, or bodybuilder becomes easily discouraged because gains in muscle mass and strength are not as dynamic as they might desire or expect. Keep in mind that everyone is not capable of running a sub-four minute mile, or a nine second hundred yard dash, or bench pressing 300 pounds. However, regardless of body type, arm length, points of insertion, etc., everyone has the capability of significantly increasing muscle strength. Due to anatomical differences, people will respond to the same exercise program differently. Therefore, the efforts or results achieved by two different individuals are not really comparable or meaningful. Analyze both your assets and limitations and realize you may not be capable of developing a massive body. Do not be misled by anyone. Follow a program designed to enable you to reach **your** potential.

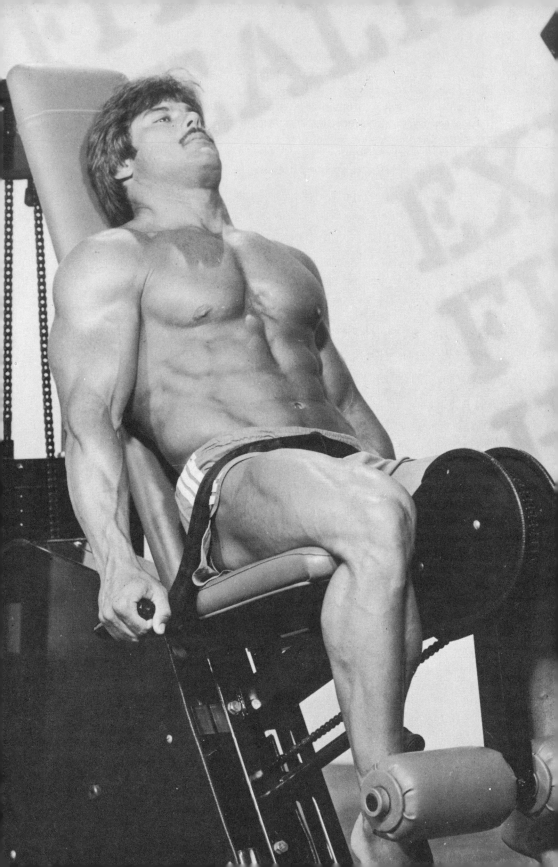

6

STRENGTH TRAINING PRINCIPLES

by
Ellington Darden, Ph.D.
Director of Research
Nautilus Sports/Medical Industries, Inc.

Proper strength training will benefit any athlete, young or old. As a result, he will be stronger, faster, more flexible, more enduring, and far less likely to suffer injury.

Muscular strength is one of the most important factors to an athlete.

Why? Primarily, because it provides the power behind every movement. Secondly, because of the role it plays in protecting the athlete from injury. Not only do stronger muscles enable an athlete to run faster, throw and kick farther, and move more efficiently; but they also provide increased joint stability—whether it be the ankle, knee, hip, shoulder, neck, elbow, or wrist.

Many high school, college, and professional athletic teams have strength training programs of some form or fashion. The results that are gained, however, from this vast amount of training time and effort fall far short of what they should be. Most athletes lightly scratch the surface of the potentially great value of strength training. The problems seem to stem from **faulty training techniques**, techniques that not only limit the results, but contribute to injuries...and a **lack of understanding** built on a long list of handed down myths and superstitions.

What is the right way to build strength? How often should you train? Which methods should you use? What exercises are best? And, generally speaking, how can you distinguish between fact and folly?

This chapter was written to answer these questions and provide you with some basic guidelines for use in establishing sound strength training programs. Six basic principles of strength training will be discussed. Following each principle are sub-principles which in turn are followed by the implications of these guidelines. I might add that these guidelines can be used with Nautilus, Universal, or conventional equipment.

1.0 **Strength training must be progressive; you should constantly attempt to increase the repetitions or resistance in every workout.**

Strength cannot be increased by the mere repetition of things that are already easy. You must constantly attempt the momentarily impossible. Attempting the momentarily impossible causes the body to resort to its reserve ability. Forcing the body to use this reserve ability is an important factor in stimulating a muscle to get stronger.

Sub-principle 1.1　In general, best results will occur if repetitions are kept in the 8 to 12 range.

If you perform less than 6 repetitions of an exercise, little inroads will be made into your reserve ability. On the other hand, if you perform over 15 repetitions, you will probably fail from a lack of oxygen, rather than from having reached a point of actual muscular failure. Once again you would not be working inside the level of your reserve ability. Greater inroads can be made into your reserve ability, if you work with resistance you can handle from 8 to 12 repetitions.

Sub-principle 1.2　When you perform 12 repetitions—or more—that is the signal to increase the resistance (by approximately 5%) in that exercise at the time of the next workout.

Empirical evidence has shown that optimum strength gains for the skeletal muscles occur when the exercise is at least 40 seconds in duration, but not more than about 70 seconds. Therefore, if you performed 10 repetitions of a given exercise, simple division reveals that each repetition should take from four to seven seconds.

Sub-principle 1.3　Never terminate a set simply because a certain number of repetitions have been completed; a set is properly finished only when additional movement is utterly impossible.

Under ideal conditions, your progress should be steady and consistent. Most training, however, does not take place under ideal conditions. As a result, strength increases are often up and down. For example, over a two-week period of time, the number of strict repetitions that you perform of a curl with a 100-pound barbell might look like the following: 8, 8, 9, 11, 10, 13. Regardless of the guide number of repetitions you're attempting to perform, you should curl until you cannot bend your arms. But, you should only record the number of repetitions you performed in perfect form.

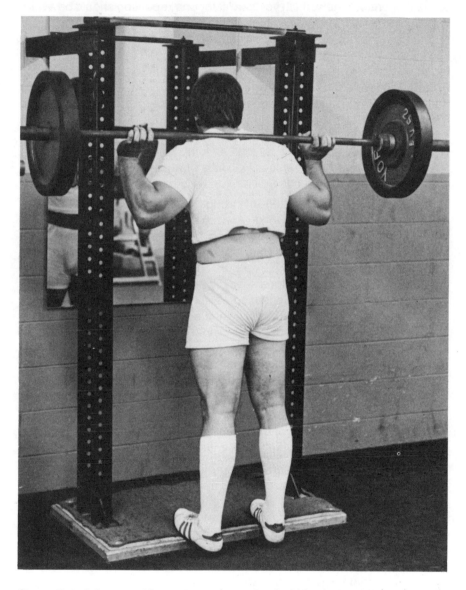

Strength training must be progressive; you should constantly attempt to increase the repetitions or resistance in every workout.

Sub-principle 1.4 Training should be done to build strength, not demonstrate it; therefore, how much you can lift for one repetition should be avoided.

Lifting maximum weights, as in weight lifting, certainly requires strength. But it also requires skill, a skill that must be developed by the practice of lifting maximum weights, and a skill that is of no value for any other purpose except lifting weights (competitive weight lifting). In fact, this skill is actually dangerous. Why? Because it exposes the muscles and connective tissue to a level of force that may cause injury. An injury will result when the forces involved in suddenly lifting (or more correctly, "throwing") a weight exceed the structural integrity of a muscle, tendon, or joint. All the worthwhile results of strength training can be produced with little or no risk of injury by using 8 to 12 repetitions in each exercise.

Implications. The cornerstone of strength training is progression, or constantly trying to increase the workload each training session. The only practical way to be progressive is by using barbells, dumbbells, or weight machines (e.g., Universal and Nautilus).

It is important to keep accurate records on your progress. The weight and the number of perfect repetitions should be written down immediately after each exercise. Also the time spent on each workout should be recorded.

Best results are usually produced when a set involves at least 8 repetitions and not more than 12 repetitions. Single repetition, maximum possible attempts, should be avoided at all costs...unless you're a competitive weight lifter. If you're not willing to perform actually progressive exercise (and it is certainly not an easy style of training), then you will never produce the final results that could have been produced.

2.0 The building of strength is related to the intensity of exercise: the higher the intensity, the better the muscles are stimulated.

Working men commonly perform enormous amounts of work, with very little in the way of strength increases as a result of their efforts. Careful research has established the cause and effect relationship involved in this situation; greatly increased muscular strength is not produced by common labor because the intensity of muscular contraction is low.

The "overload principle" is required for the production of significant increases in muscular strength. The muscles must be exposed to a load that produces high-intensity contraction.

Intensity of contraction has probably been best defined as percentage of momentary ability. When a muscle is producing as much pulling force as it is momentarily capable of doing, then maximum intensity of contraction is involved.

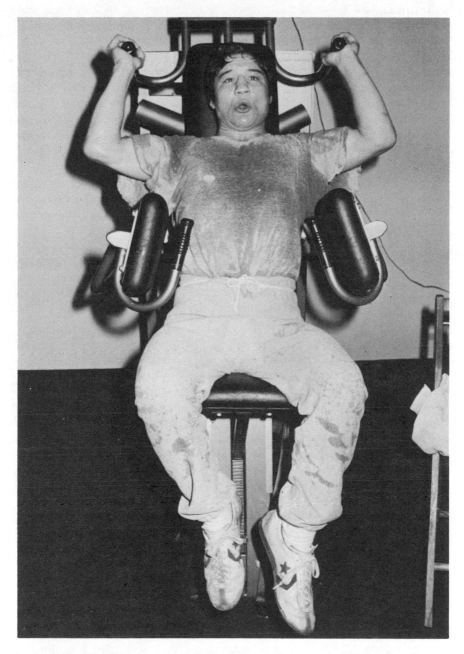

The building of strength is related to the intensity of exercise: the higher the intensity, the better the muscles are stimulated.

Sub-principle 2.1 Individual muscle fibers perform on an "all or nothing" basis; only the number of fibers that are actually required to move a particular amount of resistance are involved in any movement.

In effect, a fiber is working as hard as possible—or not at all. A movement against light resistance does not involve a small amount of work on the part of all of the fibers in the muscles contributing to this movement. Instead, only a few fibers are involved—the minimum number of fibers that are required to move the imposed resistance—and the remainder of the fibers are not involved. But the fibers that are working, are working as hard as possible—as hard as possible at that moment.

One individual fiber may be involved in each of several repetitions in a set of an exercise, but it will not contribute an equal amount of power to each repetition. The fiber will always be working as hard as possible—or not at all—but its strength will decline with each additional repetition.

Thus, in practice, a set might involve a number of fibers in much the following fashion. The first repetition involves 10 fibers, with each fiber contributing 10 "units of power" to the movement. The second repetition involves the same 10 fibers, which then contribute only 9 units of power each, and one previously uninvolved fiber (an eleventh fiber, a fresh fiber) that contributes 10 units of power, bringing the total power production up to the same level as that involved in the first repetition. The third repetition might involve the same initially used 10 fibers, with each of them now contributing only 8.1 units of power, plus the eleventh fiber that was used previously only during the second repetition, and which now contibutes 9 units of power, plus a twelfth fiber, a fresh fiber that is involved for the first time only during the third repetition and contributes 10 units of power.

Each of the first three repetitions, therefore, would result in exactly the same amount of power production. And all of the involved fibers would always be contributing to the limit of their momentary ability. The fibers, however, would not be contributing equally, and the actual number of involved fibers would change from repetition to repetition.

If the set was ended at that point, then little or nothing in the way of growth stimulating was produced—because none of the fibers was worked very hard, and because there were still unused fibers in reserve.

In order to produce significant growth stimulation, the set must be continued to a point where as many as possible of the available fibers have been involved—and where at least some of the fibers have been worked to a point of total failure.

Sub-principle 2.2 A set that is terminated prior to the point of failure will not involve the maximum available muscle fibers.

Sub-principle 2.3   A slight decrease in the intensity of effort will cause a disproportionate reduction in the results.

Sub-principle 2.4   It is impossible to measure intensity of effort less than maximum possible (100%) effort.

Exercise below a certain percentile of the momentary existing level of ability will produce no increases in muscular size and strength, regardless of the amount of exercise. There seems to be a definite "break-over" point, a point below which growth will not be stimulated, and above which growth will be stimulated. Having passed above that break-over point in the required intensity of exercise, the results seem to increase in a geometric fashion.

It may be that somewhat less than 100% of the momentary possible level of intensity is all that is required to produce maximum growth stimulation. But even if that might be the case, it is obvious that any such difference in the required intensity of effort and an outright 100% intensity of effort is of no significance.

And even if it was proven that all that was required for maximum possible growth stimulating was a level of intensity of, for example, 95% of momentary ability, just how would you propose to use such information? How would you actually know if you were working at a level of 95%, instead of 90%, or 85%? How would you measure it?

But you can measure 100%, simply by performing each exercise to a point of utter failure.

Sub-principle 2.5   In order to obtain maximum possible intensity of exercise, you must be closely supervised and "pushed."

If left to their own devices, most people will not train properly. Human nature being as it is, all of us (to a greater or lesser extent) will both consciously and unconsciously do almost everything possible to make an exercise easier. Observe any group of athletes training without supervision and you will see all types of "cheating" movements mixed in with a consistent "stopping short of failure." Exercise should be made harder, not easier—and when you make exercise harder, it must be properly supervised—every repetition of every exercise of every workout.

Implications. High intensity of muscular contraction is the single most important factor in exercises performed for the purpose of increasing muscular strength. It is very easy to slip back into a much easier style of training, frequently without being aware that you are doing so. Therefore, for maximum possible results, someone that knows what they're doing should supervise each of your workouts.

3.0 Each repetition should be performed with special attention given to a slow speed of movement, a great range of movement, and pre-stretching of the involved muscles.

Sub-principle 3.1   The speed of movement must not be too fast and not too slow.

If you performed a barbell exercise at various speeds while standing on a force plate connected to a recorder, you could clearly see the difference between slow and fast repetitions. Repetitions performed in a slow, smooth manner apply steady force throughout the entire movement. Fast repetitions apply force to only a small portion (at the start and at the end) of the movement.

Sub-principle 3.2   Special attention should be given to the lowering portion (eccentric contraction) of all exercises.

Research has shown that for building muscular strength, lowering the resistance is more important than raising the resistance. A good rule of thumb is...it should take 2 seconds to raise a weight and 4 seconds (or twice as long) to lower the same weight. All in all, it should take about one minute to complete a set of 10 repetitions.

Sub-principle 3.3   "Jerky" movements should be avoided at all costs.

When a weight is jerked or thrown, a large amount of force (usually from three to four times the actual weight) is directed on the muscles and joints. This is both dangerous and unproductive.

Sub-principle 3.4   The range of movement of each repetition should be as great as possible (from full extension to full contraction).

In order to contract, a muscle must produce movement. And in order to contract fully, a muscle must produce a full range of possible movement. If the movement resulting from muscular contraction is less than full range, then the entire length of the muscle is not involved in the work. In addition, prevention of injury is most likely where the muscles have been strengthened in every position and over a full range of possible movement.

Sub-principle 3.5   Each repetition should start from a pre-stretched position.

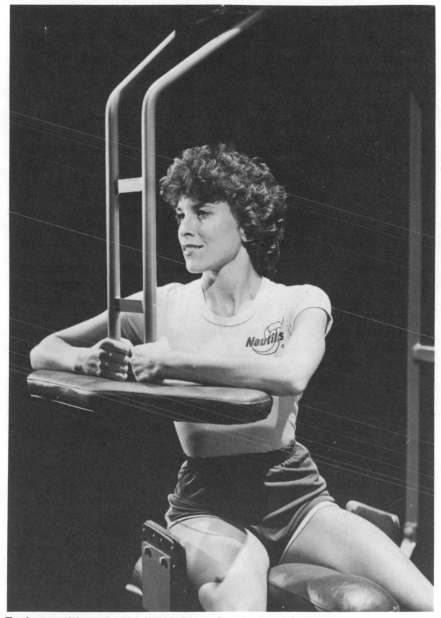

Each repetition should be performed with special attention given to slow speed of movement, a great range of movement, and pre-stretching of the involved muscles.

Pre-stretching is involved when a relaxed muscle is pulled into a position of increased tension prior to the start of contraction. Pre-stretching, properly applied, enables you to handle heavier weights and thus bring into action a greater percentage of your muscle mass during each repetition. For example, the weight should be lowered from the contracted position in a controlled manner until the bar is about one inch from the position of full extension. At that point, there should be a quick "twitch." Immediately following the quick "twitch," the movement should be slowed down in a controlled manner. The only rapid manner of the bar should be during the last portion of the lowering part of the repetition and the first part of the raising part of the repetition. The remaining portion of each repetition should always be performed slowly.

Implications. Many of you are involved or have been involved in some type of strength training program. Perhaps you've always performed fast, jerky repetitions, with little attention given to the lowering portion (eccentric contraction) or the movement. It is hard to break old habits. In fact, the act of breaking these old habits means that you must reduce the resistance in almost every exercise. It is important, therefore, to understand that...**lifting a weight is not enough, regardless of the amount of weight. How you lift a weight is a factor of far greater importance.**

Remember, it should take approximately 2 seconds in the raising part and 4 seconds in the lowering part of each exercise.

There are certain things you can do to intensify the lowering portion of some exercises. Two "spotters" can assist you in lifting the weight (a much heavier weight than you could normally lift yourself) and then allow you to lower the weight in a controlled fashion. Or, in a chinning and dipping movement, you can attach a 25-pound dumbbell to a belt around your waist, step up on a chair to the top position, and lower yourself very slowly (8-10 seconds).

With Universal or Nautilus machines, you can perform the movement in a slightly different manner. Raise the resistance with two limbs, and lower with only one limb. Raise with two, lower with the opposite.

As for pre-stretching in a strength training exercise, there is a thin line between (1) pre-stretching a muscle in the starting position and following through with the repetition in the proper form, and (2) pre-stretching a muscle in the starting position and throwing the resistance. The key points to remember are pre-stretch—move quickly—and then slow down. If in doubt, always perform a repetition **slower**, rather than faster.

4.0 Exercises should be selected that involve the greatest range of movement of the major muscle groups.

First of all, a thorough mechanical analysis should be made to determine the muscle groups that are directly involved in your particular sport. Most sports require great strength in all muscle groups, with gymnastics and sprinting being possible exceptions. Once you determine the muscles that need to be strengthened, the next step is to select exercises that involve full-range movement (or as close to full-range movement as possible) for these muscles.

In order for an exercise to be full-range, there must be resistance throughout the movement, in the extended position, in the mid-range, and in the contracted position. Full-range movements are impossible with a barbell or a Universal machine in all but a few exercises: shoulder shrugs, standing calf raises, and wrist curls with the forearms on a declined surface. Full-range movements, however, are possible with a wide variety of Nautilus machines. The Nautilus machines that provide full-range exercise are as follows: hip and back, leg extension, leg curl, pullover, behind neck, rowing, double shoulder (primary movement), double chest (primary movement), neck and shoulder, 4-way neck, rotary neck, and several varieties of bicep curl and tricep extension machines.

If full-range resistance is impossible, as it will prove to be in most exercises, then select exercises that provide the greatest range of movement. For example, the full squat, stiff-legged deadlift, chin-up, parallel dip, press, and curl.

Sub-principle 4.1   Generally speaking, the greater the mass of the muscle involved, the greater the value of the exercise.

Using conventional equipment, the exercises that involve the greatest muscle mass are compound movements, or exercises that involve rotation of two or more joints. For example, the standing press (which involves movement around the elbow and shoulder joints) is a much better exercise than the tricep extension (which involves movement around the elbow).

Sub-principle 4.2   Do not try to improve a sport skill by devising a strength exercise that is similar to the skill.

This principle is the one most likely to be violated by both the experienced and inexperienced coach and athlete. An example should make this point clear.

Motor learning research indicates that learning a simple movement with a badminton racquet, such as hitting a bird against the wall, will impede the learning (negative transfer) of an apparently similar skill, hitting a tennis ball against a wall. In both skills similar stimulus conditions are present: a racquet, an object to be hit, and a wall. However, the reponses required are different. In badminton, wrist action is very important, while in tennis the wrist should remain relatively stiff.

Similarly, practice at putting a 20-pound shot will not help an athlete to improve his 16-pound shot putting ability. In fact, it will probably confuse him. Punting or passing a five-pound football would be another step in the wrong direction—of course it would help if the athlete wanted to **learn how** to punt or pass a five-pound football.

Yet, thousands of coaches have their athletes perform arm and leg strengthening exercises in a manner that stimulates a skill (e.g., bench presses performed very rapidly for improving power in swinging a baseball bat, or jumping squats with dumbbells for improving jumping ability). To practice movements that are **nearly** the same as those of the task can not only be confusing, but it can be disastrous.

How, then, should an athlete strength train? He should select exercises that **do not** simulate the skills he desires to improve—exercises that are totally different in meaning, form, and method of execution. Exercises that involve no inter-task transfer...no positive transfer...no negative transfer.

Athletes should develop strength **generally** in all major muscle groups. Then, this general strength can be used to improve any specific ability that requires the contraction and extension of the strengthened muscles.

Anyone who has ever used a barbell is aware that the exercises provided by the use of such a piece of equipment are not full-range movements. At some points in most barbell exercises, there is no resistance at all—at the start of a curl, at the end of most forms of curling, at the top position in a squat or a press of any kind. If you can "lock out" under the weight in any position, then you do not have full-range resistance. In such a case you are providing exercise for only part of the muscles that you are trying to work.

Full-range resistance can only be provided by a machine that rotates on a common axis with the body part that is moved by the muscles being worked. When this requirement is met, then it becomes possible to provide exercise that actually exceeds the range-of-movement that is possible for most trainees. At this point in time, Nautilus sports/Medical Industries makes the only exercise machines that actually provide full-range exercise. Therefore, if you have access to Nautilus machines, be sure and use them. You will get faster and better results.

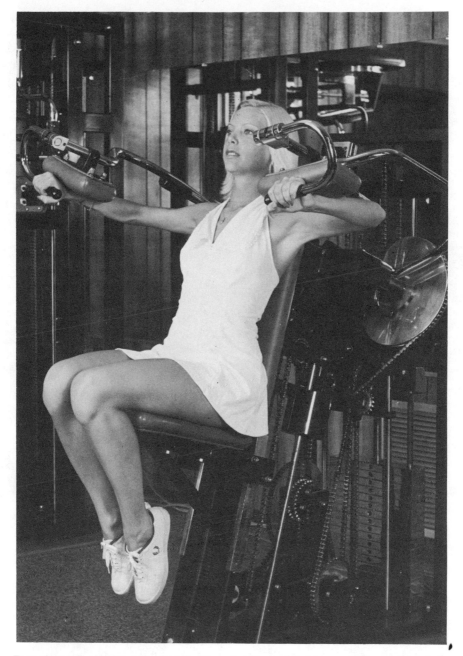

Exercises should be selected that involve the greatest range of movement of the major muscle groups.

Implications. The following exercises, grouped by muscle group and equipment, are applicable to most strength training programs:

Muscle Group	Barbells/Dumbbells	Universal Gym	Nautilus Machines
Buttocks/lower back	squat stiff-legged deadlift	leg press hyperextension	hip and back squat leg press
Quadriceps	squat	leg extension leg press	leg extension squat leg press
Hamstrings	squat	leg curl leg press	leg curl squat leg press
Calves	calf raise	toe press on leg press	calf raise on multi exercise toe press on leg press
Latissimus dorsi	bent-over rowing bent-armed pullover stiff-armed pullover	chin-up pulldown on lat machine	pullover behind neck torso/arm chin-up on multi exercise
Trapezius	shoulder shrug dumbbell shoulder shrug	shoulder shrug	neck and shoulder rowing torso

Deltoids	press press behind neck upright rowing forward raise side raise with dumbbells	seated press upright rowing	double shoulder • lateral raise • overhead press omni shoulder rowing torso
Pectoralis majors	bench press dumbbell flies	double chest parallel dip	• arm cross • decline press • parallel dip on multi exercise
Biceps	standing curl	curl chin-up	compound curl bicep curl omni curl
Triceps	tricep extension with dumbbells	press down on lat machine	compound tricep tricep extension omni tricep
Forearms	wrist curl	wrist curl	wrist curl on multi exercise
Abdominals/obliques	sit-up side bend with dumbbells	sit-up leg raise	abdominal curl leg raise on multi exercise
Neck	neck bridge (dangerous)	neck harness	4-way neck rotary neck neck and shoulder

5.0 **All workouts should begin with the largest muscle groups and proceed down to the smallest.**

Sub-principle 5.1   Greater overall strength will result if the largest muscular structures of the body are worked first.

Two reasons are primarily responsible for this sub-principle. (1) When a muscle grows in response to exercise, the entire muscular structures of the body grows to a lesser degree—even muscles that have not been exercised. Thus, the larger the muscle that is growing—or the greater the degree of growth—the greater this overall effect will be. (2) It is almost impossible to reach the required condition of momentary muscular exhaustion in a large muscle if the smaller muscle groups that serve as a link between the resistance and the large muscle groups have been previously exhausted. As a result, it is important to work the largest muscles first—while the system is still capable of working with the desired intensity.

Sub-principle 5.2   Faster rates of growth will result if growth is proportionate.

It is very common for young athletes on a strength training program to ignore the development of their legs entirely, while concentrating on their arms and muscles of the torso. On such a program, the arms will grow to a point, but then additional growth will not occur—or at least not until heavy exercises for the legs are added to the training program. Apparently having reached a maximum permissible degree of disproportionate development, the body will not permit additional arm growth until the legs are also increased in size. Therefore, for the best results from exercise, it is essential that your training program be well rounded—that some form of exercise be included for each of the major muscle masses of your body.

Implications. For best results, the order of exercise should be as follows:

- Hips and lower back
- Legs
    quadriceps
    hamstrings
    calves
- Torso
    back
    shoulders
    chest
- Arms
    triceps
    biceps
    forearms
- Abdominals
- Neck

The hips and legs have the greatest potential for developing strength and muscle mass, so they should be exercised first.

The next body segment to be exercised should be the torso. Generally speaking, when exercising the torso muscles, you should alternate a pressing movement with a pulling movement. By alternating a pressing exercise with a pulling exercise, you will allow the opposing muscles time to recover before performing another exercise.

Always work your arms after the larger and stronger muscles of the torso. To fatigue the smaller and weaker muscle groups of the arms and then perform a torso exercise would provide little benefit for the torso muscles.

When exercising the upper arm muscles (biceps or triceps), you must perform either a pulling or pressing movement. Therefore if the last exercise performed for the torso is a pressing movement (whch involves the triceps) the first exercise for the arms should be a pulling or curling movment (for the biceps), or vice versa.

The forearms should be worked after the biceps and triceps. The reason here is that your grip strength (forearm flexors) is needed to assist in the performance of the other upper body and arm exercies.

Since the abdominal muscles are used in most exercises to stabilize the rib cage and abdominal wall, these muscles should be worked after the arms. To perform high-intensity exercise for the abdominals at an earlier time in your routine would make it difficult to exert a maximum effort on an exercise to follow in which the abdominals act as stabilizers.

You should always work your neck muscles last. Why? Because if these muscles are fatigued first, you'll have a hard time performing an exercise that depends on the support of the head by the neck muscles.

Applying the above guidelines to conventional equipment or Nautilus machines, a basic workout might look as follows:

Conventional Equipment
- Squat (barbell)
- Stiff-legged deadlift (barbell)
- Leg press (leg press machine)
- Bent-armed pullover (barbell or dumbbells)
- Standing press (barbell)
- Chin-up, palms-up grip (horizontal bar)
- Shoulder shrug (dumbbells or barbell)
- Bench press (barbell)
- Standing curl (barbell)
- Dip (parallel bars)
- Sit-up (knees bent)
- Neck harness

Nautilus Machines
- Hip and Back
- Leg Extension
- Leg Press
- Leg Curl
- Pullover
- Double Shoulder
- Neck and Shoulder
- Double Chest
- Bicep/Tricep
- Ab/Ad Machine
- Abdominal Machine
- 4-Way Neck

6.0 Increases in strength are best produced by very brief and infrequent training.

Sub-principle 6.1 High-intensity training must be very brief. It is impossible to have both high-intensity exercise and a large amount of exercise.

In some fashion that is not yet understood, high-intensity work has an effect on the entire system that can be either good or bad, an effect that seldom if ever occurs as a result of low-intensity work. If high-intensity work is followed by an adequate period of rest, then muscular growth and an increase in strength will occur.

So, high intensity work is required for growth stimulation, but it must not be overdone.

Many athletes make the mistake of performing far too much exercise; too many different exercises, too many sets, too many workouts within a given period of time. When an excess amount of exercise is performed, total recovery between workouts becomes impossible; and high-intensity training then becomes equally impossible.

You can have one or the other, but not both. You can perform high-intensity exercise on a brief and infrequent basis with good results. Or you can perform long and frequent low-intensity workouts with very poor results. But you cannot perform long and frequent workouts involving a high-intensity of work. Attempting to do so will produce rapid and large-scale losses in both muscular mass and strength. In addition, it may result in total collapse.

Sub-principle 6.2 Seldom perform more than one set of any exercise in the same training session.

Sub-principle 6.3 A well-supervised, properly conducted, strength-training session should not exceed 30 minutes.

When the requirements for a productive style of high-intensity exercise are understood, it then becomes possible to select the best exercise for a particular purpose. In most cases, not more than 12 different exercises (4-6 for the lower body and 6-8 for the upper body) should be performed in any one training session. If you are "pushed" to an all-out effort in each of the 12 exercises, you will not want to do more than one set of each exercise. In fact, your body will literally "not be able to stand" more than one set.

A set of 10 repetitions performed in proper form (2 seconds on the lifting and 4 seconds on the lowering) should take around one minute to complete. Allowing about one minute between exercises, then most athletes should be able to complete 12 exercises in under 25 minutes. Actually, as the athletes work themselves into better shape, the time between exercises should be reduced. It is entirely possible for a well-conditioned athlete to go through an entire workout (12 exercises) in less than 15 minutes. A workout performed in this fashion not only develops muscular size and strength, but also a high dgree of cardio-respiratory endurance.

Sub-principle 6.4   There should be at least 48 hours rest between high-intensity workouts, but not more than 96 hours.

High-intensity exercise causes a complex chemical reaction to take place inside a muscle. If given time, the body will compensate by causing certain muscle cells to get bigger and stronger. So, high-intensity exercise is necessary in order to stimulate muscular growth; but it is not the only requirement: the stimulated muscle must be **permitted** to grow.

Research has shown that there should be approximately 48 hours between workouts. In some cases, where extremely strong athletes are training, longer periods of time (72 to 96 hours) are required. On the other hand, however, high levels of muscular size and strength start to decrease (atrophy) after about 96 hours of normal activity. So, rest between workouts is important, but not too much rest.

An every-other-day, three times per week exercise program, also seems to provide the body with the needed irregularity of training. The human body quickly grows accustomed to almost any sort of activity—and once having adapted to such activity, then no amount of practice of the same activity will provide growth stimulation. Thus it is important to provide many forms of variation in training. Variation can occur in several different ways: (1) weight and repetitions should be varied for each workout, (2) the exercises can be occasionally changed or alternated or performed in a slightly different sequence, and (3); the training days can be varied. For example, a first workout is performed on Monday, then two days later a second workout is performed on Wednesday, then two days later a third workout is performed on Friday. Thus, on Sunday, the system is expecting and is prepared for a fourth workout, but it does not come. Instead, it comes a day later, on Monday of the next week—when the body is neither expecting it nor prepared for it. This schedule of training prevents the body from falling into a "rut"—since the system is never quite able to adjust to this irregularity of training, and great growth stimulation will be produced as a direct result.

Sub-principle 6.5   An advanced trainee does not need more exercise than a beginner; he needs harder exercise and in most cases less exercise.

Beginning trainees usually show good strength gains on most types of exercise programs, even though they may perform several sets of more than 12 exercises in each training session. They are able to make this progress (at least for a while) because they are simply not strong enough to use all of their recovery ability. As they get stronger, however, they do use up all of their recovery ability—and further growth stops. The stronger the athlete becomes, the greater resistance he handles, and the greater inroads he makes into his overall recovery ability. Therefore, the advanced trainee must reduce his overall exercises (e.g., from 12 to 10) and only train in the high-intensity fashion twice a week. On Monday he might train hard, on Wednesday medium, and on Friday hard. The Wednesday workout would not stimulate growth (the workout would actually keep his muscles from atrophying), it would permit growth by not making significant inroads into the athlete's recovery ability.

Implications. During the off season, all athletes should strength train three times a week. Since most athletes interested in strength training are at a beginning or intermediate level, they should make good progress on three, high-intensity workouts a week. If their progress slows down, they should reduce the high-intensity workouts to two a week, and slightly reduce their total number of exercises. **Never** should the stronger, more advanced trainees perform multiple sets or more than 12 different exercises in any one training session.

Other conditioning drills, especially those performed in a high-intensity fashion (wrestling, sprinting, agility drills, etc.) should be kept at a minimum. Remember, you must have adequtae time (at least two days) to recover from high-intensity work.

During the season, the players need at least one high-intensity workout a week to keep the strength they have developed during the off season. Many athletes, in fact, actually increase their strength during the season by continuing to train hard twice a week. For example, they work out hard the day after a game, and take a second high-intensity workout three days later.

Over a six-month period of time, most trainees should see strength increases of from 50-100% in all the recommended exercises. How much will this added strength improve your athletic ability? Obviously, the answer will vary from athlete to athlete depending on age, prior ability, overall potential, motivation, and many other factors. But in all cases, there will be a measurable degree of improvement and this improvement will produce a level of performance that would not have been reached without proper strength training.

And what degree of protection from injury will be provided by proper strength training? Again the answer will vary; since many complex factors are involved. It should be apparent, however, that a strong limb is far less likely to be injured than a weak one, and it is well established that strength training increases not only the size and strength of muscles, but the connective tissues and even the bones.

In conclusion, the greatest benefits of strength training occur when the exercises are performed in the **proper** manner. The following rules summarize the principles that should be used in organizing a sound strength training program.

1. Select exercises that involve large muscle groups throughout a great range of movement.

2. Stress correct form; avoid fast, jerky movements.

3. Raise the weight to the count of two—lower the weight slowly and evenly while counting to four and repeat.

4. Perform only one set of 8 to 12 repetitions in all exercises.

5. Continue each exercise until no additional repetitions are possible.

6. Attempt to increase repetitions or weight whenever possible.

7. Work the largest muscles first.

8. An entire workout should include a maximum of 12 different exercises.

9. Train no more than three times a week.

10. For best results, you should be supervised and pushed throughout, every workout.

STRENGTH TRAINING—use it properly and you've got everything to gain and nothing to lose.

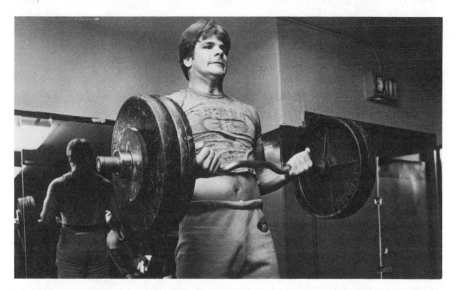

Increases in strength are best produced by very brief and infrequent training.

Bibliography

Allman, Fred L. "Prevention of Sports Injuries" *Athletic Journal* 56:74, March, 1976.

Astrand, Per-Olaf, and Rodahl, Kaare. *Textbook of Work Physiology.* New York: McGraw-Hill, 1970.

Cratty, Bryant J. *Movement Behavior and Motor Learning.* Philadelphia: Lea and Febiger, 1967.

Darden, Ellington. "What Research Says About Positive and Negative Work." *Scholastic Coach* 45:6,7, October, 1975.

DeLorme, T. L., and Watkins, A. L. "Techniques of Progressive Resistance Exercise." *Archives of Physical and Medical Rehabilitation* 29:263-273, 1948.

Goldberg, Alfred L., and others. "Mechanism of Work-Induced Hypertrophy of Skeletal Muscle." *Medicine and Science in Sports* 7:185-198, 1975.

Jokl, Ernst. "Physique and Performance." *American Corrective Therapy Journal* 27:99-114, 1973.

Jones, Arthur. "High Intensity Strength Training." *Scholastic Coach* 42:46, 47, 117, 118, May, 1973.

Jones, Arthur. *Nautilus Training Principles,* Bulletins #1 and #2. DeLand, Florida: Nautilus Sports/Medical Industries, 1970.

Komi, P. V., and Buskirk, E. R. "Effect of Eccentric and Concentric Muscle Conditioning on Tension and Electrical Activity of Human Muscle." *Ergonomics* 15:417-434, 1972.

Lamb, Lawrence E. "Exercise, Muscles." *The Health Letter* 1:#9, 1973.

Larson, Leonard A. *Fitness, Health, and Work Capacity.* New York: MacMillan, 1974.

Peterson, James A. "Total Conditioning: A Case Study." *Athletic Journal* 56:40-55, September, 1975.

Sandow, A. "Excitation-Contraction Coupling in Skeletal Muscle." *Pharmacology Review* 17:265, 1965.

7

STRENGTH TRAINING FUNDAMENTALS AND TECHNIQUES

by
Daniel P. Riley
Washington Redskins

The first requirement for an effective weight training program is to learn the basic skills and guidelines attendant to a properly conducted strength development program. Adhering to these fundamental precepts will enable you to accomplish two objectives: (1) to be able to train in as safe a manner as is possible; and (2) to maximize your gains in muscular development.

WARM-UP

Although contradictory information exists regarding the possible benefits of warming-up or limbering-up before training with weights, common sense dictates that some energy should be devoted to a warm-up period if for no other than safety reasons. Since warming-up increases the internal temperature of your body which in turn affects the elasticity and extensibility of the involved muscle tissue, warming-up before engaging in rigorous activity is generally believed to make you less prone to muscle pulls, tears, etc. The length of the warm-up period and the activities to be followed depend on the individual. For most individuals, five to ten minutes of limbering-up should suffice. Suggested warm-up activities include: jumping-jacks, running-in-place, and lifting light weights through the ranges of motion specific to the exercise in the weight training program.

MUSCLE SIZE AND STRENGTH

When you place a demand on your muscles, your muscles respond to the stress by growing in size, also referred to as hypertrophying. This growth is the result of an increase in the size (**not the number**) of the individual fibers and the tissue (fascia) which surrounds the fibers. The strength of a muscle is roughly proportional to its cross-sectional area. All other factors being equal, the larger the muscle, the stronger the muscle.

MUSCLE SORENESS

In the initial stages of a properly conducted strength training program, you exert tension on infrequently used or unused muscle fibers. This tension causes waste products (specifically lactic acid and carbon dioxide) to accumulate faster than your body can use or remove them. These waste products are believed to bring about the feeling of soreness by sensitizing local pain receptors. The best method for relieving muscle soreness and stiffness is to train for three or four successive days at a level of normal workout intensity. After this initial conditioning stage, all muscle soreness should disappear. Any subsequent introduction of new movements in the training program will result in some soreness. Temporary relief of muscle soreness can be achieved by applying heat and massage to the affected muscles in order to speed up circulation, thereby abetting the removal of the aforementioned waste products.

PROPER TRAINING TECHNIQUES

A complete mastery of the basic techniques of strength training is a critical factor in the degree of success you can achieve in a strength training program. Without total adherence to the correct techniques, the exercises will not be performed properly; you cannot capitalize on your existing potential for improvement; and your susceptibility to injury is increased. You should become **totally familiar** with the basic techniques for performing each exercise which are described in detail in Chapters 11-14. If you are lifting weights for the first time, you should devote the first several workouts to practicing the basic movements involved in each exercise with relatively light resistance in order to gain a working familiarity of the proper techniques.

SPOTTERS

Spotters are individuals who assist someone engaged in lifting weights. This assistance may be before, during, or after the completion of an exercise. A spotter has two primary responsibilities: (1) Prevent injuries to either the lifter or anyone in the adjacent vicinity, and (2) assist the lifter in such a way as to facilitate the proper execution of the exercises (e.g., bring a heavy weight into the starting position for an exercise).

A spotter can also aid you by providing constant verbal feedback. Such feedback can stimulate your desire to achieve an "all-out effort" by discouraging you from quitting when the pain and discomfort becomes almost unbearable. Verbal encouragement also helps reinforce proper training techniques. Frequently, as you become more fatigued, your adherence to correct form will gradually decrease unless you are told to perform otherwise. In negative only training, the spotter will often assume additional major responsibilities.

The guidelines for serving as a spotter are basic. During most exercises, come from beneath the weight (not over it) in order to prevent the weight from falling on the lifter. Remember that the last repetition, if performed properly, has a substantial effect on the degree of improvement achieved by the lifter. Allow the lifter to do as much work as possible on the final repetition. A final note—**NO ONE** should assume the responsibilities of a spotter unless he/she is aware of the proper spotting techniques.

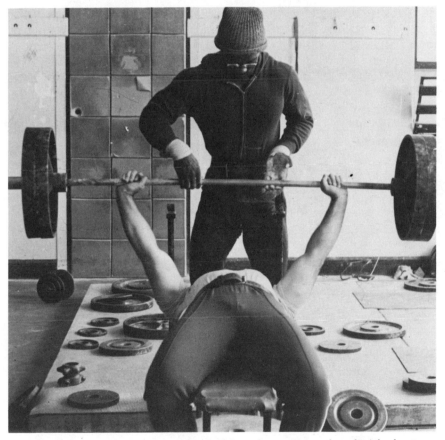

No one should assume the responsibilities of a spotter unless he/she is aware of the proper spotting techniques.

BREATHING

While strength training you should synchronize your breathing with the exercise. There is a physiological need for breathing during each and every repetition of any exercise. Adherence to the proper breathing pattern facilitates the function and efficiency of an exercise. The most consistent and efficient method for breathing properly is to inhale whenever the resistance is being lowered or pulled toward your body and exhale when the resistance moves away from your body (e.g., blow the weight away from your body).

You should never hold your breath while training. On occasion, inexperienced lifters may hold their breath in order to "gut out" an extra repetition. More often than not, this practice results in a decrease in the efficiency of the exercise. In addition, holding your breath while training can also produce either dizziness or unconsciousness. This results from the buildup of inner thoracic (inner rib cage) pressure due to the great pressure or force of the weight on your body when you are holding your breath. This pressure, built up inside the rib cage, compresses the right side of the heart which in turn restricts the flow of blood, and consequently O_2 to your entire body. Some exercises bring on the symptoms of the Valsalva Phenomenon more readily than others (i.e., squat, seated or military press, deadlift, biceps curl, bench press).

SAFETY CONSIDERATIONS

If you adhere to proper lifting techniques and utilize a reasonable level of common sense, strength lifting is a relatively safe activity. Most injuries result from either carelessness or ignorance. The following guidelines should be followed:

- Never train with weights at a high level of intensity without having mastered the techniques involved in performing the exercise.
- Use spotters whenever necessary.
- Always make sure that plate collars for the free weights are securely tightened.
- Wear footwear in order to cushion the blow from a falling object and to avoid stubbing the toes.
- When loading or unloading one side of a barbell, load or unload the other side evenly.
- Remember that the weight room is not a playroom. Be considerate of others.

RUBBER SWEAT SUITS

Perspiring is your body's mechanism for preventing overheating. When the temperature of your body rises, the perspiration process begins. Evaporation of perspiration cools your body's surface which in turn helps control

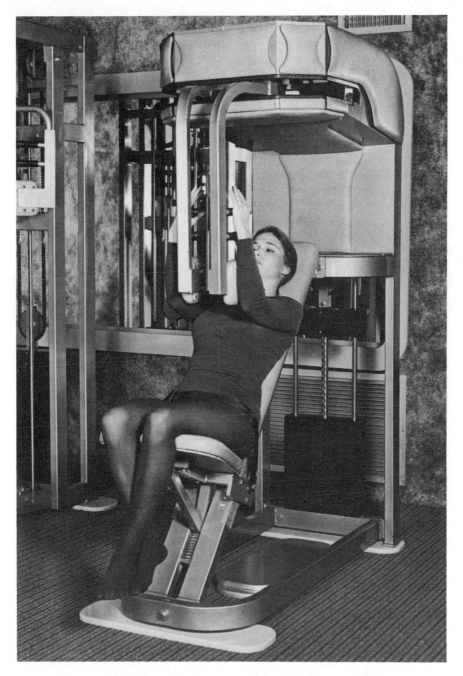

You should never hold your breath while training.

body temperature. Covering your body with a plastic or rubber sweat suit prevents the natural cooling down process of the body to take place. The heat produced is not dissipated, and the temperature of the body continues to rise. This causes a rise in blood pressure and overtaxes your heart. Simply stated, these suits serve no practical purpose in a strength training program (or any other properly conducted conditioning program for that matter).

EXERCISE ANTAGONISTS

Pairs of muscle groups which oppose each other are called antagonists (e.g., the biceps and the triceps). Practically every muscle in your body has an antagonist. To develop one muscle or group of muscles upsets the equilibrium of the opposing muscles. As a muscle becomes stronger than its antagonist, the flexibility of the joint controlled by the affected musculature is decreased. As a result, both the joint and the involved muscles are more susceptible to injury.

Many individuals are frequently guilty of not achieving a balance of strength in opposing muscle groups. Such individuals can be seen, for example, exercising the quadriceps by running hills, stadium steps, riding bicycles, etc., but ignoring the hamstrings. This leads to a loss in both flexibilty and strength in the hamstrings (in relation to their quadriceps) and leaves their hamstrings more susceptible to pulls and tears.

Another muscle group which is often over-developed is the pectorals (chest muscles). If you exercise only your chest muscles, and not the antagonist (upper back muscles), your pectorals become stronger than the muscles of your upper back. The muscles of your chest then gradually pull the shoulder girdle forward which may cause a condition known as "round shouldered". As a result, when developing a weight training program, you should always include an exercise for the antagonist of all muscles developed by your program.

EXERCISE THROUGH A FULL RANGE OF MOVEMENT

Flexibility, one of the primary components of physical fitness, is defined as the capacity of a joint to move through a full range of movement. The primary factor affecting that capacity is the musculature surrounding the joint. When the joint is periodically required to go through a full range of motion, the involved muscles retain their natural elasticity. When a joint is not utilized through its full range of movement on a regular basis, the surrounding musculature tends to tighten up, causing it to lose some of its elasticity. As a result, the joint becomes less flexible. For athletes, the loss of flexibility can

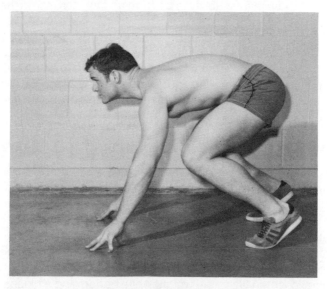

Figure 7-1. Football player's stance.

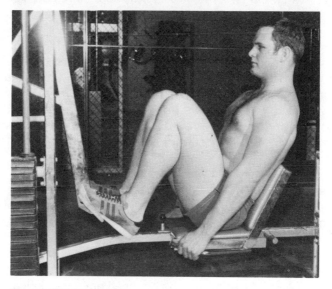

Figure 7-2. Leg press.

Figures 7-1 and 7-2 illustrate the close relationship between the flexibility required for a specific sport's task (football player's stance) and the range of motion involved in the proper execution of a specific strength training exercise (leg press).

result in a decrease in their ability to perform and an increase in the chances of being injured.

Contrary to superstition and unfounded myths, properly performed strength training exercises actually increase flexibility. In fact, exercising through a full range of movement makes it impossible to decrease your flexibility. Adhering to correct lifting techniques will enable you to develop strength throughout the entire range of movement for your body's musculature.

POSITIVE VERSUS NEGATIVE WORK

Two distinctive movements can be observed when you are performing a strength training exercise: The raising of the weight and the lowering of the weight. The raising of the weight is considered positive work and the lowering of the weight negative work. When performing positive work, the muscle is shortening (contracting). While lowering the weight the muscle is lengthened. The muscles used to raise the weight are the same muscles used to lower the weight.

For example, when lifting the weight while performing a biceps curl, your muscles are performing work while they are shortening. When the weight is lowered, the same muscle group is performing the work. In this instance, however, your biceps are lengthening.

The negative portion of an exercise is just as important as the positive movement. Unfortunately, negative work is often ignored by individuals engaged in strength training. Since it is easier for you to lower than to raise that same weight, the tendency is to be less conscious of form when you are lowering the weight. Both movements, however, should be performed as exacting as possible, perhaps placing even a greater emphasis on the lowering of the weight. It should take almost twice as long to lower the weight than it did to raise it.

Many individuals "throw" a weight rather than allow the muscles to lift it. They generate enough momentum so that the exercise becomes a ballistic movement. The body will recruit fewer fibers to perform this kind of exercise. "Throwing" the weight can be observed in many exercises but it is particularly obvious in an exercise such as the leg extension.

When raising a weight, you should control the weight's speed of movement. You should be able to stop the weight at any time during the "positive" movement. The weight should not be bounced or jerked during any part of the range of movement for an exercise.

EMPHASIS ON NEGATIVE WORK

In the previous section, it was stated that the negative portion of the exercise is as important (and some researchers believe it is more important) as the positive part of the exercise. When performing an exercise to the point of momentary muscular failure, you will eventually fail during the positive portion of the exercise. That is to say, you will reach a point where you will no longer be capable of "raising" the weight through the full range of movement. When this point has been reached, you have generally obtained maximum benefit from this portion of the program. A muscle, however, is capable of lowering much more weight than it can raise. Even though your muscles have failed during the positive portion of the exercise, they could continue to perform additional negative work. The point of momentary muscular failure for the negative portion of the exercise is much greater than for the positive movement. Therefore, you have not maximized your potential for gain from an exercise when you quit at the point when a weight can no longer be lifted through the positive phase. The only way to obtain the maximum benefits from the negative portion of the exercise is to periodically take your muscles to the point of momentary muscular failure during the negative portion of the exercise. To accomplish this, you should perform some type of training that will place an emphasis on the negative part of the exercise.

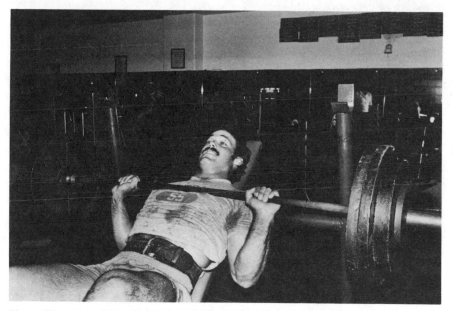

You will never reach your potential if you quit exercising at the point when you can no longer perform just the positive phase of an exercise.

There are two techniques that can be utilized to perform this function. These techniques are negative only training and negative accentuated training.

When performing negative only exercise, you engage only in the negative portion of the exercise. In short, you only lower the weight. To perform negative only exercise, you need either spotters to raise the weight for you or equipment that is specifically designed for negative only training.

The following guidelines for performing negative only training are recommended. You should use as much resistance as possible so that:

- At any point during repetitions 1-4, you can stop the descent of the resistance and momentarily change direction.
- At any point during repetitions 5-8, you can stop the descent of the resistance and pause momentarily but are unable to change direction.
- During repetitions 9 and 10, you are unable to momentarily stop the descent of the resistance.

Negative only exercise can be of great value to you if you lack the requisite muscular development to properly perform a particular exercise. For example, if you can only perform 2 pullups, it will take you a great deal of time before you are capable of performing 2-1/4, 2-1/2, 3, 3-1/4 etc. In general, two or three complete repetitions of any exercise are not enough to stimulate maximum gains in muscular development. In this instance, however, you could continue to develop muscular fitness by performing negative only pullups. By continuing to lower your body weight after you are no longer capable of performing the positive portion of the pullup, you will be strengthening the same muscles used to raise your body weight.

It is very difficult to perform some exercises in the negative only fashion, since either specially designed equipment or several spotters would be needed to raise the weight for you. Another technique which can be used to emphasize the negative part of the exercise is the "negative accentuated" method of exercising.

During negative accentuated exercise, you lift the weight with two appendages and lower it with one. Obviously, it is very difficult to perform negative accentuated exercise without the use of either a Nautilus or a Universal machine.

Negative accentuated training has many advantages. If, for example, you could perform an exercise in normal fashion at a level of 10 repetitions with 100 pounds, you would be able to substantially increase the resistance on a single limb by exercising in a negative accentuated fashion. That is to say, by raising the weight with two hands and lowering it with one, you can double the amount of resistance placed on a single limb. For example, if you lift 100 pounds with two hands on your first repetition, you would lower 100

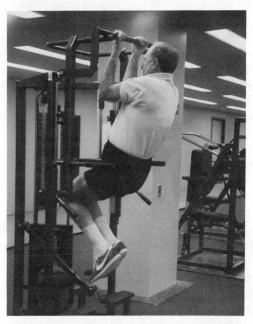

Techniques for performing negative-only chinups.

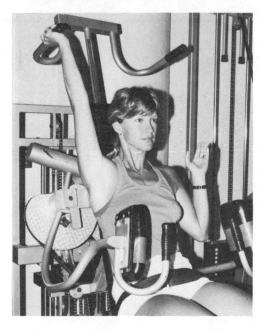

Techniques for performing a negative-accentuated exercise.

pounds with your right hand and then would alternate and lower the weight on the next repetition with your left hand. By definition, negative accentuated exercise "accentuates" the negative portion of the exercise. This type of training allows you to approach the point of momentary muscular failure during the negative portion of the exercise. It is still possible to experience momentary muscular failure during the raising of the weight (positive phase of the lift) while performing negative accentuated exercise.

The following guidelines for performing negative accentuated exercises are recommended:

- Use as much weight as possible so that you fail somewhere between 8-12 repetitions. One repetition constitutes the raising of the weight in both arms or legs then lowering it in one arm or leg.
- Eliminate all bouncing or jerking movements when making the transfer of weight from two appendages to one.
- The non-working arm or leg should be ready to immediately initiate the raising of the weight as soon as the resistance has been completely lowered.

The table below illustrates that there are advantages to performing all three methods of training (normal, negative only, and negative accentuated).

	NORMAL EXERCISE	NEGATIVE ONLY EXERCISE	NEGATIVE ACCENTUATED EXERCISE
Intensity during the positive portion of the exercise	Maximum	Non-Existent	Maximum
Intensity during the negative portion of the exercise	Moderate	Maximum	Moderately High

Table 7-1. Intensity during three types of training in both the positive phase and the negative phase.

In order to obtain the best of what each type of training has to offer and to minimize tedium in the training, I strongly recommend that you vary the methods of training you employ in your strength training program.

INTENSITY

Within safety considerations, the higher the level of intensity you reach in a strength training program the greater the results you will achieve. The level of intensity is determined by three factors: (1) the effort extended by you; (2) the use of proper training methods and techniques; and (3) the equipment used in the conditioning program.

The effort that is extended is the most important of these three elements. The greater the effort you extend, the higher the intensity of the exercise. The effort being extended reaches its maximum when you reach the point of momentary muscle failure. That is, you train to a point where the muscle being exercised has failed momentarily and can no longer execute another properly performed repetition. For example, while performing the squatting exercise, you will eventually reach a point when you can no longer recover from the squatting position to the starting position (standing). A 100% effort has not been achieved by you if you do not reach the point of momentary muscular failure.

Equipment that varies the resistance is essential for maximum muscle fiber recruitment throughout the entire range of movement. Since such equipment varies the resistance to accommodate the various strength curves of your body, the recruitment of muscle fibers is greater. Regardless of the equipment being used, a maximum effort must be extended and all the proper training techniques must be observed to achieve high level intensity and maximum gains in muscular development.

If you are interested in training at a level of high intensity, you should make an attempt to experience high intensity exercise in order to evaluate your present conditioning program. In most instances, you may be simply unaware of what constitutes a high intensity effort. Frankly, it is almost impossible when training alone to reach the point of momentary muscular failure. The use of a training partner is the most effective method if you want to push yourself to your physical (and sometimes psychological) limits.

You should remember that there is a minimum level of intensity at which you can train and still continue to improve your level of muscular devlopment. Although you can train at a point past the minimum required level and achieve gains, you should keep in mind that a less than maximum effort will produce less than maximum results.

GRIPS

There are four grips that can be used when performing the various barbell exercises. These grips are the overhand, the underhand, the alternate, and the false grip.

● The **overhand grip** is the most widely used grip when performing the barbell exercises. The thumbs are hooked underneath the bar with the knuckles placed on top of the bar.

● When the **underhand grip** is used, the thumbs are hooked above the bar and the knuckles are placed underneath the bar.

● When using the **alternate grip**, a combination of the overhand and the underhand grip is used. One hand is placed above and one hand below the bar. The alternate grip is the strongest grip of the four. It can be used when performing an exercise similar to the deadlift or shoulder shrug.

● When using the **false grip** the thumbs are not hooked around the bar. It is a grip that should not be used by a novice lifter. It can be a substitute for the overhand or underhand grip when performing certain exercises. It is often substituted because it is a more comfortable grip. However, as its name implies it is not a very safe grip.

The width of the particular grip being used varies with the individual and the exercise being performed. The width of the grip should provide the following: maximum range of movement; isolation of the specific muscle or group of muscles being exercised; and comfort.

The grip should be consistent when performing the same exercise. For example, each and every time you perform a bench press, you should use the same width grip.

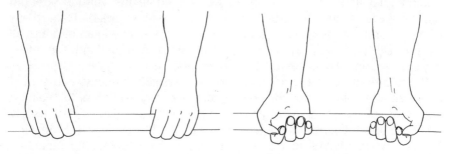

Overhand grip.   **Underhand grip.**

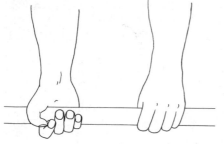

Alternate grip.   **False grip.**

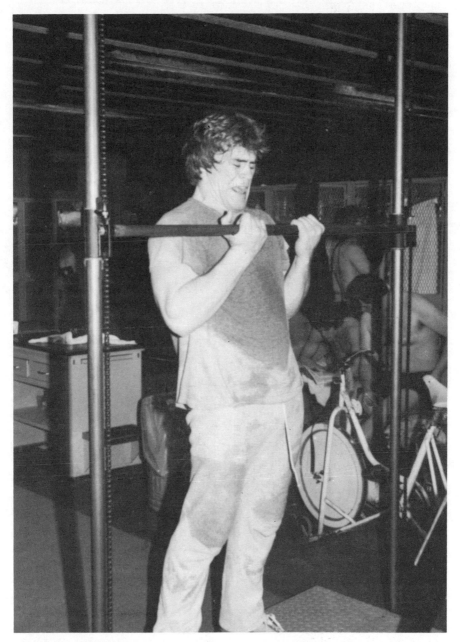

Within safety limitations, the higher the level of intensity you reach in a strength training program, the greater the results you will achieve.

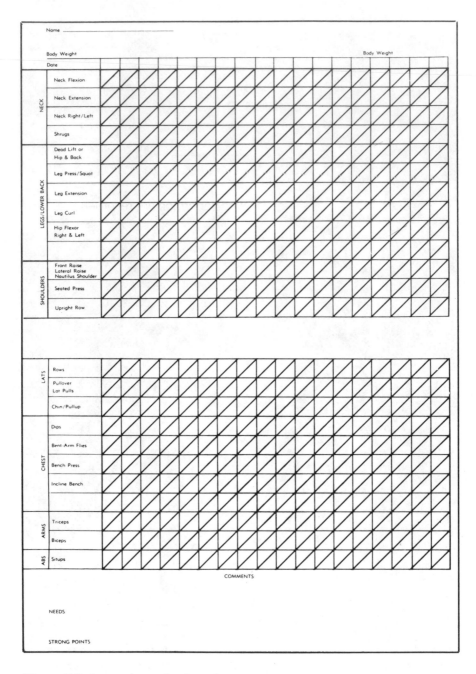

Figure 7-3. A sample workout card.

RECORD WORKOUT DATA

During each workout, the amount of resistance lifted and the number of repetitions performed for each exercise should be recorded. This recording helps eliminate the duplication of a previous workout and provides incentive for improvement. Since during a single workout you will frequently perform many exercises at varying repetitions and workloads, it will be quite difficult to recall from one workout to another the specific accomplishments of prior training sessions. As a result, unless you keep a record of all workout data, the danger exists that you will not make the regular program adjustments which are necessary for self-improvement. Figure 7-3 provides an example of a typical workout card. Note that the date of the training session, the exercise in the program, the amount of resistance for each exercise, and the number of repetitions each exercise was performed are recorded.

Recording workout data also provides you with an incentive for increasing the amount of resistance or the number of repetitions you can perform on each exercise. If for example, you performed 8 repetitions using 100 pounds of a particular exercise on your last workout, your goal should now be to try and perform at least 9 repetitions with that same weight.

A record of workout data can also serve as a measuring stick for improvement. As such, it can serve as an invaluable tool for anyone who wants to monitor the performance of someone in the weight room. As a general rule, you should strive for a certain degree of continual progress in muscular development. The gradual improvement in performance in the weight training room often serves as a stimulant for maintaining a personal commitment to the conditioning program. Eventually, you will receive more substantial feedback from your conditioning efforts in the form of looking and feeling better.

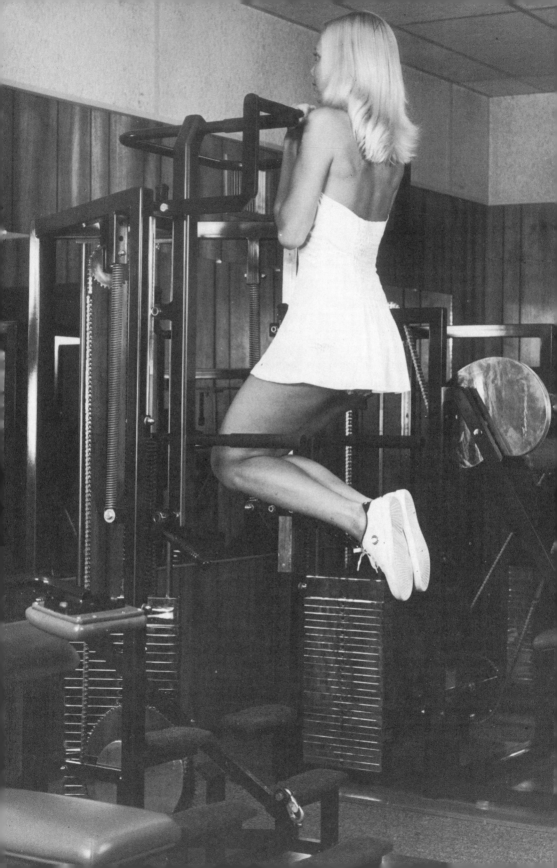

8

HOW TO ORGANIZE A STRENGTH TRAINING PROGRAM

by
Daniel P. Riley
Washington Redskins

Everyone who wants to develop muscular fitness should engage in a strength training program that "produces the best results," "consumes the least amount of time," and "best prepares the athlete to perform in his specific athletic event." The methods used to organize a program for strength training should focus on and accomplish these objectives.

The methods I recommend for organizing your strength training program are the most demanding methods available. They are also the most productive. If you fail to reach your potential using these methods, don't blame the program. These methods have been proven conclusively.

To effectively organize a strength training program, you should focus on eight variables. They include the following:

- How many repetitions?
- How much weight?
- How many sets?
- At what level of intensity?
- How much rest between exercises?
- Which exercises?
- In what order should the exercises be performed?
- How often should the workouts be performed?

HOW MANY REPS?

I recommend that you use 7-12 repetitions as a guideline. Perform at least 7 reps, but not more than 12. Remember that these are just guidelines. You can perform fewer than 7 reps or more than 12 reps and get stronger. However, best results will be obtained when 7-12 reps are performed.

More important than the number of reps performed is the length of time each exercise is continued. Muscles do not count reps. They accumulate time. Best results have been observed when an exercise is continued for at least 40 seconds but not more than 70 seconds.

HOW MUCH WEIGHT?

For **maximum** gains, a weight should be selected that will cause you to experience momentary failure between 7 and 12 reps. The first time you perform an exercise, you must select a starting weight. If you have never performed the exercise before, you will have almost no idea how much weight with which to start.

The first step must be to learn how to perform each exercise. There is a specific skill required to perform each exercise and you must learn that skill before progressing to a heavier weight. Initially, you should choose a weight at which you can very easily perform 10-12 reps. Once you feel relatively comfortable performing the exercise, you should then carefully progress to an effective training weight.

What is an effective training weight? A weight is "effective" when it is heavy enough to overload your muscles adequately to cause an increase in your strength. It may take several workouts to find this weight. Do not rush the process of progressing from the starting weight to an effective weight. This may invite possible injury. On the other hand, do not procrastinate. Three to five training sessions should be more than adequate. Until an effective weight is being lifted, you will not gain any strength from your efforts.

The amount of weight used and the number of reps performed should be recorded on a workout card. This will eliminate reproducing an effort already exerted in a previous workout.

When should you add more weight? As soon as you can properly perform 9 or 10 reps, use a weight that forces your muscles to fail on the 9th or 10th rep. Once you can complete a 9th or 10th rep, add more weight.

How much weight should be added once you can perform 9 or 10 reps? It will depend upon the exercise, the equipment, and how long you have been training. During the first few weeks of training the amount of weight used will increase significantly. Five to ten pound increases aren't unusual. As the weeks pass, the increments will gradually become smaller. Add as much weight as possible for each exercise every workout. Too much weight has been added if you cannot perform at least 7 reps.

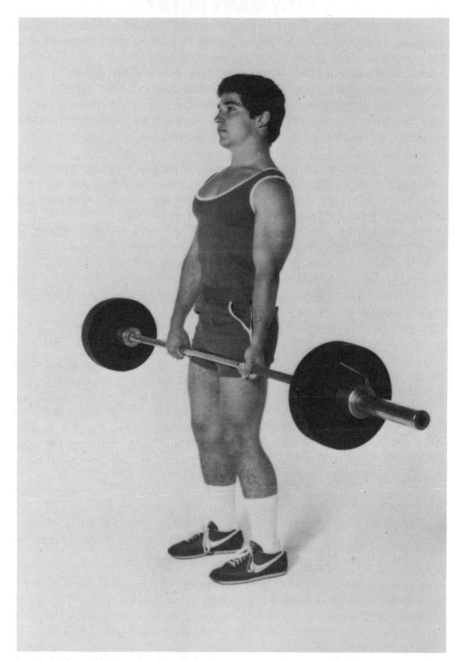

A weight is "effective" when it is heavy enough to overload your muscles adequately to produce an increase in your strength.

HOW MANY SETS?

A set consists of the total number of repetitions executed each time an exercise is performed. For example, you do 10 push-ups and then rest. You have performed one set of 10 reps of the push-up exercise.

One set of push-ups, or any other exercise, is all that is required to stimulate **maximum** gains in strength, size, and endurance. Traditionally, many people believe that multiple sets are required to produce the best results. If you perform more than one set, however, you did not perform the first set properly. You will not want to perform a second set if the first one is performed correctly.

There is a specific skill required by a training partner or spotter to help you use these methods. For best results, you must be disciplined and willing to tolerate relatively high levels of muscular discomfort. These two factors limit the results obtained in many strength training programs.

You should remember that if you want to perform a second (or third, or fourth) set:

- You didn't exert an all-out effort on the first set.
- Your training partner doesn't know how to properly spot for you.

Everyone has physical assets and limitations. Realistically, few individuals have the ability to make truly outstanding gains. If you do not develop to your potential, do not blame the number of sets being performed as the problem.

At one time or another, I've seen almost every combination of sets and reps possibly used. I'm convinced that one set **will** produce maximum gains. Some individuals might claim they've tried using only one set and didn't observe great results. You can assume that these individuals were not performing the one set in the recommended manner. It's obvious that they lack the knowledge and skill needed to effectively implement the recommended methods. It's easier for some people to fault the proper techniques than to admit they lack the expertise.

If for whatever reason you perform more than one set, you should follow the same guidelines for each set as if you were doing only a single set. Each set should be terminated at the point of muscular exhaustion. Do not stop on a given set simply because you've completed a certain number of reps.

LEVEL OF INTENSITY

Intensity is something very difficult to describe. A training partner with the right skills can teach you the true meaning of intensity in a hurry. The higher the intensity of exercise, the more productive the exercise. If the intensity of an exercise drops below a certain level, it will cease to be productive.

As the intensity of exercise increases, the amount of exercise performed must decrease. If the intensity of exercise is as high as it should be, you can only perform one set. It is difficult and almost impossible to measure any-

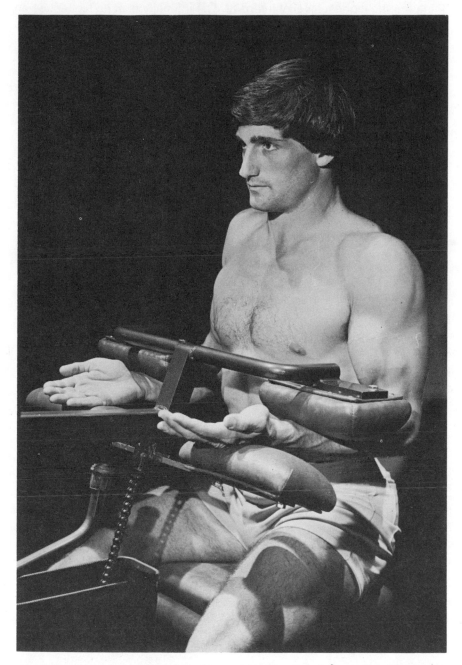

One set of any exercise is all that is required to stimulate maximum gains in strength, endurance, and muscular size.

thing but the highest level of intensity. The intensity is at its highest when you have reached momentary muscular failure. If you've never experienced high intensity exercise, try running up a steep hill. Run as hard as possible. In just a short period, your legs will fatigue to the point where you cannot move them or even hold up your own body weight. You literally collapse to the ground. In this instance, your muscles have temporarily reached the point of failure. Momentarily (for just a few seconds), they have failed. They will recover quickly and soon you could get up and run again.

In the weight room the same phenomenon should occur. You should fail with the intensity as high as it can be for at least 40 seconds but not more than 70 seconds. It will be extremely difficult to perform each exercise in this manner. You'll recover quickly once you adapt to this style of training. Don't be tempted to perform an additional set. It won't produce better results, and it could become counterproductive.

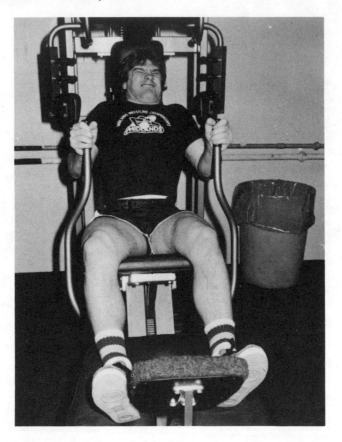

The intensity of an exercise is at its highest when you have reached the point of momentary muscular failure.

REST BETWEEN EXERCISES

The amount of time taken from the completion of one exercise until you begin the next exercise is considered the **rest interval**. You should move from one exercise to the next, allowing little or no time to rest between exercises. This style of training will consume the least amount of time. Strength training may only be a small part of your overall conditioning program. There may be many other demands on your time that may be far more important.

The less time you spend in the weight room, the more time you will have to do other things. The bodybuilder and weightlifter find great pleasure in spending hours in the weight room. In a typical workout, they can be observed performing an exercise and then spending a significant amount of time resting before performing the next exercise. More time is spent resting and chatting between exercises than is spent actually working out.

There are several options that you have while working out that will conserve time yet allow for periods of adequate rest. You can perform an exercise with your training partner providing the supervision. Upon completing the exercise, you can reverse roles and become the spotter. You can now supervise your training partner through the same exercise. This procedure can continue throughout the entire routine. Another alternative would be to perform an entire series of exercises and then supervise your training partner through the same sequence of exercises.

WHICH EXERCISES?

Which exercises you perform will be almost totally dictated by the equipment you have available. The equipment **will not** affect the results you obtain. **How** you use the equipment you have is the critical factor.

You should strengthen each of the major muscle groups in your body. From the equipment available, you should select an exercise to develop each major muscle group. If more than one type of equipment is available, then use it. There are both advantages and disadvantages to all the equipment on the market today. If possible, I recommend adding variety to your program by using all of the equipment you have available. Performing similar exercises on different types and pieces of equipment may help you to prevent boredom mentally and physically.

The shoulder muscles can be used as an example. You might ask, "What exercises can I do to develop my shoulders?" The side lateral raise is one of several exercises that will develop your shoulder. The side lateral raise can be performed with dumbbells, manually, or with a Nautilus machine. It's the same exercise with different equipment. The muscles don't know what type of equipment you're using. If you adhere to the proper techniques with each type of equipment, you'll develop similar results.

To simplify the process of identifying which exercises to perform, I suggest that you divide your body into five major segments: the neck, the lower body, the upper body, the arms, and the abdominals. With the equipment you have available, perform 3-5 exercises for the neck, 4-6 for the lower body (to include the lower back), 4-6 for the upper body, 1-2 for the arms, and 1 for the abdominals. Excluding the neck, you should perform between 10 and 13 exercises in a workout.

ORDER OF EXERCISE

There are two general guidelines that can be used to determine what the order of the exercises should be:

- Exercise the priority muscle groups first.
- Whenever possible, attempt to alternate pushing and pulling movements for the muscles of the upper body and arms.

There are no magical exercises that can be performed. There is no special order of exercises. General guidelines can be used, but this is one area where a wide latitude exists. Some athletic events, however, require particular attention to certain areas of the body. For example, wrestlers and football players risk injury to their necks. Therefore, athletes in these sports should perform exercises for the neck near the beginning of their workouts. If neck exercises were performed at the end of their workouts, there may be a tendency for them to place less emphasis on this part of their body. It's obvious that the neck should not be neglected.

The muscles of your hips, legs, and lower back are the major muscles used to perform most vigorous (athletic) tasks. I recommend that exercises for these areas be emphasized early in your workout. As a general rule of thumb, exercises for the major body segments should be performed in the following order:

● Neck		● Hips, legs, lower back
● Hips, legs, lower back		● Neck
● Upper body	**or**	● Upper body
● Arms		● Arms
● Abdominals		● Abdominals

While exercising the muscles of your upper body and arms, try to alternate pushing and pulling movements. The chest, shoulders, and triceps are the primary muscles used to perform any pushing movement (i.e., bench press, seated press, dips). The position of your body can be changed to place the emphasis more on one muscle group than another (i.e., bench press-chest, seated press-shoulders). The primary muscles used to perform any pulling movement are the lats and biceps (i.e., seated row, lat pulldown, bent over row).

To allow adequate recovery time between exercises (without allowing time to rest), you should perform a pushing movement (i.e., dip) and then a pulling movement (chin-up) whenever possible. This is not a hard and fast rule but a recommended guideline.

While exercising each body segment (i.e., upper body), try to periodically change the order in which you perform the exercises. You should **not** perform the same exercises in the same order workout after workout. You will quickly become bored both mentally and physically. For example, assume that your program includes the following five exercises:

- bench press
- chin-up
- dip
- bent over row
- seated press

During your workouts, you should periodically change the order of the exercises. Many different combinations of these exercises exist. For example:

• dip	• seated press	• bench press
• chin-up	• chin-up	• bent over row
• bench press (or)	• bench press (or)	• seated press
• bent over row	• bent over row	• chin-up
• seated press	• dip	• dip

Frankly, there is no special order of exercises, and you shouldn't believe that there is. Variety can also be added to your program by performing different exercises for the same muscle group. For example, instead of the bench press, perform the incline or decline press. Instead of the squat, perform the leg press.

One guideline that you should follow is to exercise your arms after exercising the stronger and larger muscles of your torso. The arms are used to perform most upper body exercises. Your arm muscles are smaller and weaker than the stronger muscles of your torso. If biceps curls were performed before chin-ups, the chin-up exercise would be adversely affected by doing curls first. However, the biceps will not be adversely affected if chins are performed before curls.

If possible, try to keep the order of exercises within these body segments: neck, lower body, upper body, arms, abdominals. Within each of the major body segments, you should vary the order of exercises as much as possible.

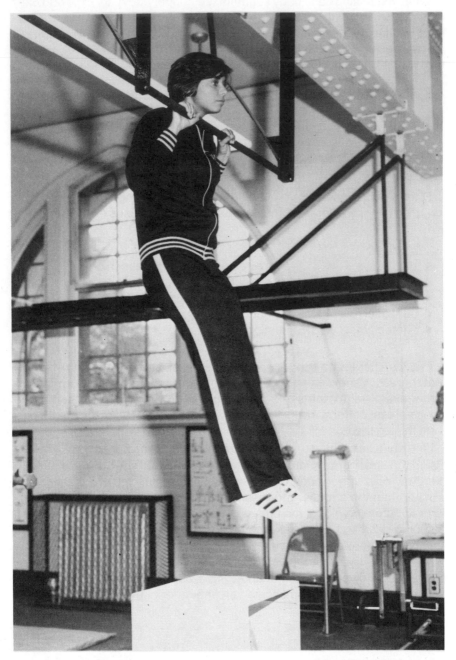

A muscle needs 48-72 hours to recover from the stresses imposed upon it during a strength training workout.

FREQUENCY OF WORKOUTS

If you are an athlete, you should train three times a week (i.e., Mon.-Wed.-Fri.) during the off-season and at least twice a week during the season. For the in-season program, I suggest that you work out the day after a game and again at least 48 hours before the next game. If you are not an athlete, but merely someone who wants to stay in top shape, I recommend that you work out three times a week on alternating days.

You must give your body a chance to recover from the demands of the lifting. Currently, the literature indicates that a muscle needs approximately 48 to 72 hours to recover from an effective amount of exercise. If too much exercise is performed in a workout, you may not maximally recover in a 48-72 hour period.

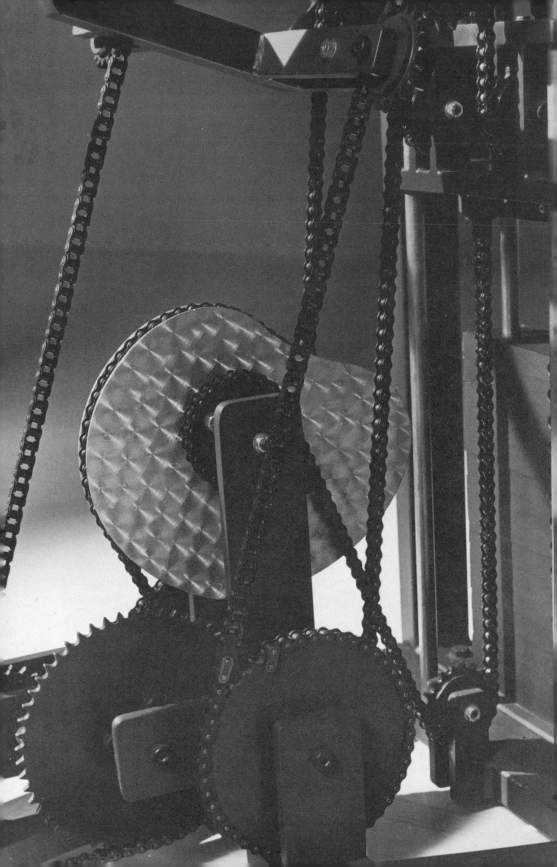

9

STRENGTH TRAINING EQUIPMENT

by
Daniel P. Riley
Washington Redskins

Few people are fortunate enough to have a wide variety of equipment available from which to initiate and continue their strength development program. If more than one type of equipment is available, you should use the equipment that will best meet your needs. When making this selection, the primary considerations should be availability and personal preference. The equipment used for strength training should be readily accessible with the least amount of inconvenience (compatible to your workout schedule, least amount of travel, etc.)

The most important consideration you face when making a decision on what type of equipment to use is really personal preference. Remember that it is the **quality** of training (not the type of equipment) that is the critical factor in producing the greatest increases in muscle strength and mass. Significant gains in strength can be obtained by using any kind of equipment that will overload your muscles.

In ancient Greece, Milo of Crotona significantly increased his strength by hoisting a baby bull on his shoulders daily. As the time passed, the bull matured and gradually grew heavier. Milo continued to hoist the animal which allowed his body to gradually adapt to the additional stress. As a result his body grew stronger and stronger.

This was probably the first recording of the overload principle being observed. Milo of Crotona did not have either modern technology or a variety of weight training equipment. Yet, he was able to significantly increase his strength simply by making the muscles work harder each time he trained.

The best equipment in the world will not increase your strength if it is not used properly. Should a choice of equipment be available, list the advantages and disadvantages of each and subjectively make a decision. Depending upon your needs and interests, it may be desirable to incorporate more than one type of equipment into your strength development program.

Refrain, however, from falling prey to the various assortment of gimmicks guaranteed to increase strength and muscle mass in a very short period of time. The only way to significantly increase both strength and muscle mass, regardless of the equipment used, is hard work based on sound training principles—and, it will take time.

Each piece of strength training equipment has its advantages and disadvantages. In this chapter the advantages of the most common and widely-used types of equipment available, including conventional free weight equipment, the Universal gym, and isokinetic machines, are presented. The Nautilus machines and Nautilus training concepts are discussed in Chapters 13 and 14.

FREE WEIGHT EQUIPMENT

The basic equipment necessary for a strength training program using conventional free weight equipment includes:

- **Barbell:** The term barbell refers to a bar 5 to 7 feet in length. The diameter and weight of the bar may vary. Collars are used to secure the barbell plates to the barbell. Figure 9-1 illustrates both the fixed and adjustable collar. The advantages of the fixed collar are:
  a. The plates will not slip off while exercising.
  b. The plates, if secured to the bar, will not be scattered about the weight room.
  c. You do not have to adjust the weight (saves time).
  d. The primary advantage of the adjustable collars is that weight can be added or subtracted if desired.

The barbell shown in Figure 9-2 is an Olympic barbell. The calibrated Olympic bar weighs 45 pounds and is approximately 87 inches long. The bar was designed for use in the Olympic Games to perform Olympic lifts. Some of the advantages of the Olympic barbell are:
  a. It is used universally.
  b. Its length provides a whipping action.
  c. Rotating sleeves prevent weight plates from sticking to the bar.

When lifting heavy weights, you will find that an Olympic bar will bend significantly. While lifting a weight, the bending of the bar can provide a "whipping action" which assists the lifter. The rotating sleeves, which are located on both ends of the Olympic bar, allow the weight plates to rotate without affecting the lifters' grip on the bar. The Olympic barbell plates are much larger in diameter than the conventional barbell plates. This prevents the Olympic bar from falling on and crushing the Olympic lifter should he/she fall while trying to raise the weight upward and overhead. Olympic collars weigh 5 pounds each.

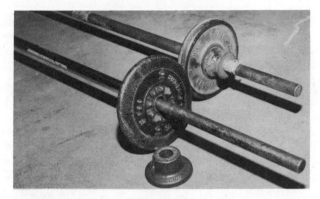

Figure 9-1

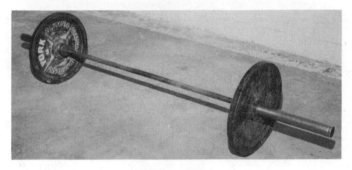

Figure 9-2

● **Dumbbell:** The term dumbbell is used to describe a short bar (8-14 inches in length) in which weight plates may be secured to both ends. A dumbbell can be held in one hand to perform many of the exercises that can be performed with a barbell.

The advantages of using the dumbbell are:

a. Strengthening both sides of the body equally.
b. There are some exercises that can be performed with a dumbbell that cannot be performed with a barbell (side lateral raises).
c. Develop skill and coordination with both hands.
d. Adds variety to your program.
e. One arm may be immobilized by a sling or cast, but exercises can still be performed with the uninjured limb with a dumbbell.

When not in use, the dumbbells (Figure 9-3) and barbells (Figure 9-4) should be replaced or stored in racks. Plate racks (Figure 9-5) are used to store barbell plates not being used. When these racks are not used, the strength development facility becomes disorganized and unattractive. Most facilities require lifters to replace all equipment immediately after use.

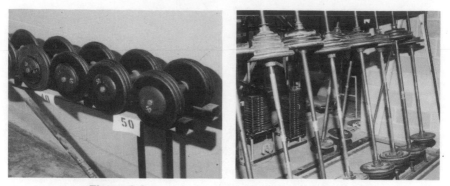

Figure 9-3
Figure 9-4

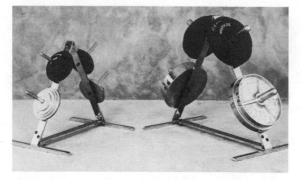

Figure 9-5

• **Curl Bar:** The shape of the curl bar (Figure 9-6) is designed to specific-ally increase the efficiency of the biceps curl exercise. The curl bar places the hands and biceps into a position that is most conducive to performing the biceps curl exercise (Figure 9-7). Many people complain of pain in their forearms (forearm splints) when performing the biceps curl with a straight bar. A straight barbell may place the hands in a position in which a great deal of strain is placed on the forearm muscles (which in turn may cause pain and discomfort).

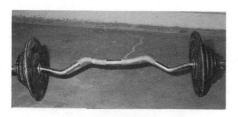

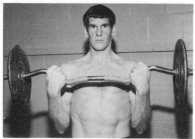

Figure 9-6
Figure 9-7

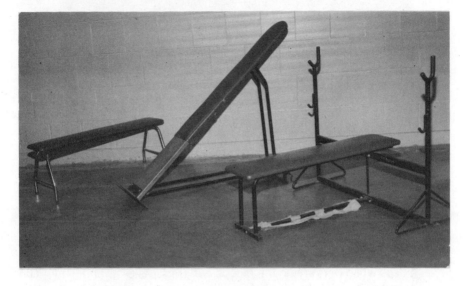

Figure 9-8

- **Benches:** Figure 9-8 illustrates some of the various types of benches on which exercises may be performed. The purpose of these various benches is to change the position of your body so that a particular muscle or group of muscles can be isolated or exercised at a specific angle.
  a. **Power Bench:** The power bench is primarily used to perform the bench press exercise. The bench press is one of the power lifts, which is where the power bench derived its name.
  b. **Incline Bench:** The standard incline bench rests at a 45° angle. The purpose of the incline bench is to place your body into a position which is midway between the position assumed to perform a bench press and a standing military press. The incline press will, therefore, place the demand on the upper pectoral region and the anterior (front) region of the deltoids.
  c. **Decline Bench:** A standard decline bench was designed to place your body into a position so that the demand is placed on the lower region of the pectorals when the decline bench press is performed. Figure 9-9 illustrates a decline bench.
  d. **Multi-Purpose Bench:** The multi-purpose bench was designed to provide you with a bench on which most exercises may be performed.

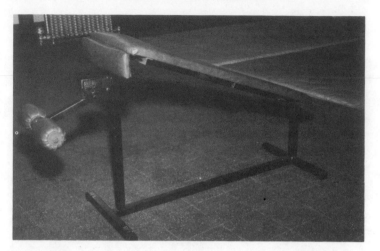

Figure 9-9

e. **Preacher Bench:** The preacher bench was designed to isolate the biceps while performing the biceps curl (Figures 9-10 and 9-11). The preacher bench helps to minimize "cheating" or improperly performing the biceps curl. The disadvantage of the preacher bench is that the biceps do not have resistance on them in the contracted position.

f. **Abdominal Board:** The abdominal board is designed to place your body into positions in which the demand is directed on your abdominal muscles.

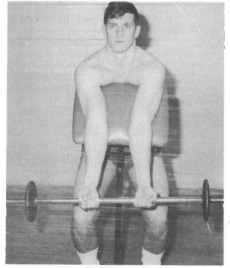

Figure 9-10

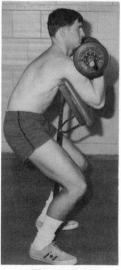

Figure 9-11

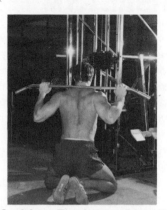

Figure 9-12

g. **Lat Machine:** The lat machine (Figure 9-12) was designed to effectively isolate your latissimus dorsi muscles. In addition, the lat machine may be used to perform a variety of exercises for some of the other muscle groups in the body.

h. **Lifting Platform:** The purpose of the lifting platform (Figure 9-13) is to prevent damage to the floor when performing specific exercises requiring overhead lifts.

i. **Squat Racks:** Squat racks are utilized to perform the squatting exercise with a barbell. Heavy weights are used to perform the squatting exercise. The squat racks allow you to initiate the exercise with the barbell across your shoulders. Most lifters are normally not capable of lifting the weight from the floor to the shoulders.

j. **Leg Extension-Leg Curl Machine:** The leg extension machine is used to effectively isolate your quadriceps while performing the leg extension exercise. The same machine may also be used to perform the leg curl exercise which strengthens the hamstrings.

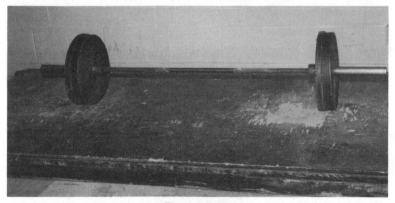

Figure 9-13

THE UNIVERSAL GYM

The Universal Gym is a unit of equipment composed of various exercise stations that can accommodate many individuals at one time (Figure 9-14). A very versatile piece of equipment, the Universal Gym is capable of duplicating most barbell exercises. It also provides the capability of performing many exercises that cannot be done with either a barbell or a dumbbell.

The Universal Gym was a primary catalyst in the widespread acceptance of strength training at the high school level. This was primarily due to the following reasons:

● The Universal Gym eliminates many of the safety hazards that exist with the barbell.

● The unit, although capable of accommodating many individuals, requires very little floor space.

● Adjustable weight stacks facilitate the changing of weights which conserves a great deal of time when many individuals are training simultaneously.

● The weight stacks travel up and down on fixed runners which reduces the level of skill and technique needed to perform the same exercise with a barbell.

● The Universal Gym is easy and uncomplicated to understand and operate.

● The entire unit can be moved by one person.

● The newest of the Universal machines offers variable resistance to accommodate to the strength curves of your muscles.

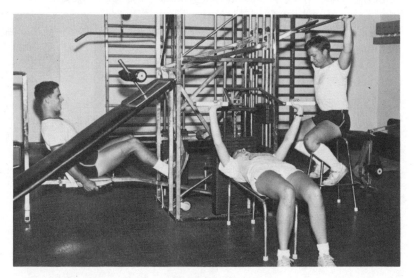

Figure 9-14

ISOKINETIC MACHINES

An isokinetic machine varies the resistance throughout a muscle's entire range of movement. When you apply a maximum effort, the isokinetic machine automatically varies the resistance to accommodate to any mechanical advantage of your body.

One isokinetic machine varies the resistance through the use of a hydraulic clutch. This phenomenon can be observed on the Mini Gym leg extension machine (Figure 9-15). Another isokinetic machine (Figure 9-16) varies the resistance by the use of cylinders filled with fluid (dash pot theory).

Some of the many advantages of the isokinetic machines are:

● The speed of movement is retarded which eliminates the use of momentum to assist in the raising of the weight (the harder the push or pull, the greater the resistance offered).

● The isokinetic machine automatically varies the resistance to accommodate the mechanical advantages of your body.

● The muscles are exerting a maximum effort each and every repetition regardless if it is the first or tenth repetition.

● The machine automatically adjusts to fatigue or pain which provides for maximum strength gains during rehabilitation.

● The isokinetic machine eliminates the use of bulky weights.

● The isokinetic unit eliminates the time needed to adjust weights.

● Muscle or joint soreness is not experienced due to the lack of eccentric contractions.

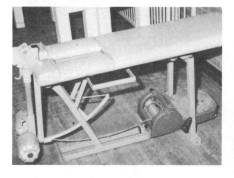

Figure 9-15

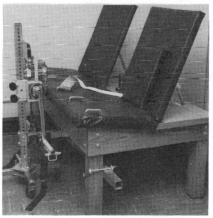

Figure 9-16

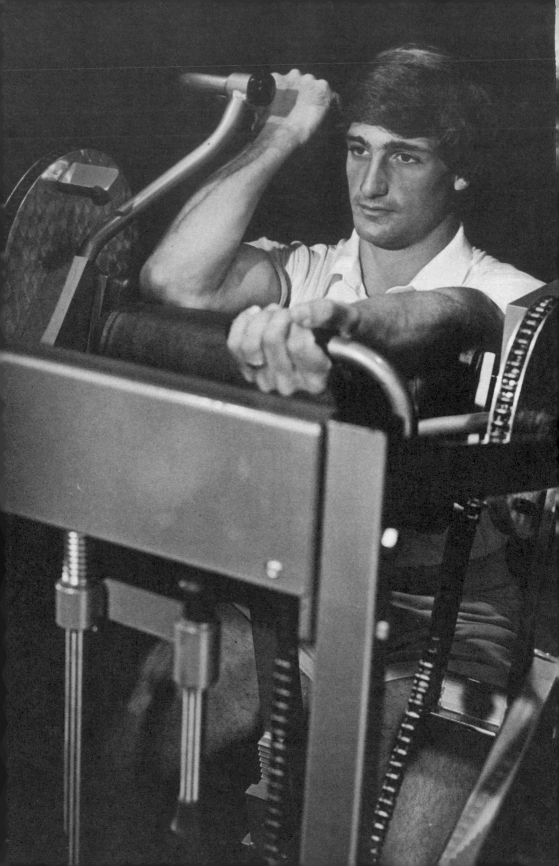

10

HOW TO PERFORM A STRENGTH TRAINING EXERCISE

by
Daniel P. Riley
Washington Redskins

The key to any strength building program is what happens during the execution of each exercise. It is what takes place between the first and last repetition of each exercise that produces the results.

To be sure, there are differences between and among the various types of equipment. Remember, it's not the equipment that produces the results. The actual stimulus for strength gains is provided by the execution of each exercise.

It doesn't make any difference if a program is recommended by a famous coach or athlete. To tell a coach or an athlete that the Washington Redskins, for example, do three sets of ten reps is meaningless. How each rep is executed is important. How each exercise is performed is the critical factor.

You should be concerned with performing an exercise in a manner that produces the best results, in the least amount of time, while best preparing yourself to be able to do the things that you like to do as safely and as well as possible.

I'm not stating that the methods described in this chapter are the only techniques that can be used to perform an exercise. Frankly, it's possible to produce increases in strength by doing almost anything which places a demand on your musculature. If, however, you want to develop maximal strength in the least amount of time and in the safest manner possible, nothing is more effective or efficient than the steps outlined in this chapter.

While performing any exercise in which a resistance is raised and lowered, you should observe the five checkpoints of a properly performed exercise. By strictly adhering to these five checkpoints, you can be assured of maximum gains without risking injury.

FIVE CHECKPOINTS

- Full range exercise
- Eliminate any fast, sudden, or jerky movements
- Emphasize the lowering of the weight
- Overload the muscles properly
- Supervision

CHECKPOINT #1: FULL RANGE EXERCISE

Full range exercise implies that the resistance should be raised and lowered through the fullest range of movement that each exercise provides. This will allow your muscles to be maximally developed through their full range of motion. Your level of flexibiity will be maintained and improved with full range exercises.

This checkpoint is based on both logic and common sense. And yet, in the typical weight room, you can see lifters violating Checkpoint #1 constantly. Why? Why would a person fail to perform an exercise properly—through the full range of motion provided? The answer is pure and simple. It's easier. By compromising the requirements of an exercise, more weight can be used, and more reps can be performed.

By using the parallel dip exercise as an example, you can observe the proper execution of a single repetition of the dip exercise (Figures 10-1 and 10-2). Note the stretched position (Figure 10-2). Your muscles are mechanically weakest in this position. It would be easier for you to stop before reaching the stretched position (Figure 10-3). It would be to your mechanical advantage. As a result, you could perform more reps. However, the additional reps would be at the expense of maximally developing your muscles at each position through their full range of movement.

You must be concerned with developing and transferring strength, not demonstrating it. When engaged in physical activity, you don't know when or where an injury may occur. Your muscles must be strengthened as much as possible through their fullest range in order to reduce the chances of you being injured while exerting yourself physically.

Whenever possible, you should make an exercise more difficult to perform. Don't make it easier by not going through the full range of motion.

Point: Raise and lower the weight through the fullest range of motion provided by each exercise.

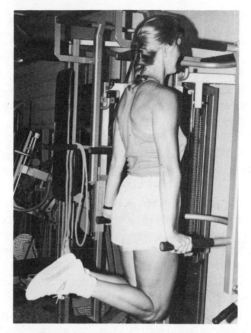

Figure 10-1. The starting position for the dip exercise.

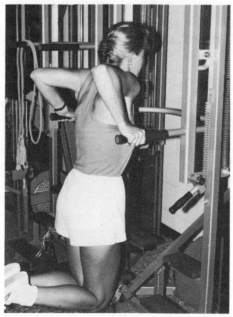

Figure 10-2. The mid-range position for the dip exercise.

CHECKPOINT #2: ELIMINATE ANY FAST OR JERKY MOVEMENTS WHILE RAISING A WEIGHT

Allow your muscles, and only your muscles, to raise the weight. You ask, "What else would raise the weight if my muscles didn't raise it?" Momentum! If you raise a weight too fast, momentum becomes involved. And if any momentum is used, it's obvious that your muscles have not raised the weight completely.

Your brain will only recruit those muscle fibers (motor units) that it needs to raise a weight. If a barbell weighs one hundred pounds, your brain will re- cruit only as many muscle fibers as it needs to raise the weight. No more, no less.

If a one hundred pound barbell is too heavy for you, two things will hap- pen. One, the barbell won't move. Two, if the bar is raised, you will have to "cheat" by throwing, yanking, or jerking the weight to raise it.

Let's assume you are capable of properly raising an eighty pound barbell. You can raise and lower an eighty pound barbell in good form. Now you are handed a bar weighing one hundred pounds. As has already been men- tioned, the bar will not move. Now you decide to raise the weight at all costs. You make up for the lack in your strength level (of being able to properly lift eighty pounds maximum and facing a bar that weighs one hundred pounds) with momentum.

What's the problem with this training technique? You're using more weight, aren't you? Or are you?

You're using more weight but your muscles are not raising more weight. You can brag to your friends that you've thrown one hundred pounds. You may as well put a five hundred pound bar on the floor, give it a shove, and watch it roll across the floor. At least that would be safer than yanking, jerk- ing, or throwing a weight just for the sake of raising it. You lift weights to be- come a better, more durable performer, not a more proficient yanker or thrower.

Using momentum to raise the weight will literally allow you to "move" more weight. But it will be at the risk of injury and at the expense of not letting your muscles do all of the work.

How fast should you raise the weight? Raise it as fast as you want, as long as the muscles are doing all of the work—without the aid of momentum.

How do you know if there's any momentum involved? One guideline that can be used is to pause momentarily in the contracted position when per- forming an exercise. There should be no bouncing or recoil of the weight at the transition point of the raising phase to the lowering phase. You should be able to stop and hold the resistance at the transition phase for a count of 1001 (Figure 10-3).

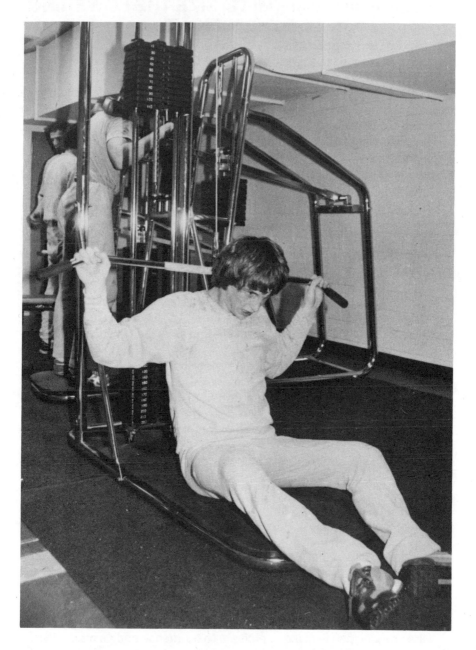

Figure 10-3. There should be no bouncing or recoil of the weight at the transition point of the raising phase to the lowering phase.

CHECKPOINT #3: EMPHASIZE THE LOWERING OF THE WEIGHT

"Can you get stronger from only raising a weight? Sure, everyone knows that. How about the lowering of the weight? Can you get stronger from only lowering a weight? Sure, I guess so, I think so. I'm not sure."

Ask the typical beginning lifter the above questions and you'll probably receive the same or similar responses. The fact is that the raising phase of an exercise is one half of the exercise. The lowering phase is the other half.

Is one more important than the other? Does one phase of an exercise produce better results than the other? To be perfectly honest, I don't really know. I do know that both the raising and lowering phase are at least equally important.

The lowering of a weight is just as productive as the raising of the weight. In fact, if I had to pick one phase as being more productive than the other, I'd have to say the lowering phase is the more important phase.

It is during the lowering phase that your muscles are stretched and pre-stretched each and every rep. Research studies support the fact that strength training maintains, and in most cases increases, flexibility.

How does this increase in flexibility occur? It can be attributed to the lowering phase of the exercise. This is the portion of the exercise where your muscles are stretched, thereby stimulating an increase in your level of flexibility.

The raising phase of an exercise is called "positive work". Your muscles are contracting concentrically. Your muscles are shortening. The lowering phase is commonly called "negative work". Your muscles are contracting eccentrically (away from the center). They are lengthening.

Why should the lowering phase be emphasized? There are at least two basic reasons:

* In any exercise, the same muscles are used to raise and lower the weight.
* Gravity.

At a minimum, the same amount of emphasis should be placed on the lowering phase because it is one half of the exercise. While doing a biceps curl, for example, your biceps raise the weight. Your biceps also lower the weight during the negative phase of a biceps curl.

Because of gravity it's much easier for you to lower a weight. It is possible for you, unfortunately, to gain little or nothing from the lowering phase of an exercise. Once you've raised the weight, you can merely allow it to fall effortlessly to the ground.

If the lowering phase of the exercise is to be intense and as productive as the raising phase, one or two things must occur.

* Take longer to lower the weight.
* Add more weight during the lowering phase.

You should allow approximately four seconds to lower the weight. Why four seconds? Remember that these are only guidelines. You should be primarily concerned with the overall amount of time spent performing each exercise. Allowing four seconds to lower the weight provides an adequate amount of time to effectively overload your muscles. Anything less than four seconds will diminish the benefits that can be obtained.

You can implement a great deal of variety into your program by varying the amount of time required to lower a weight. For example, sometimes, you can only lower the weight and take a predetermined, extended amount of time (e.g., eight, fifteen, thirty, and sixty seconds) to lower the weight. Obviously, the number of reps you perform of any given exercise will be affected by the amount of time you take to lower the weight.

With conventional exercise, you are limited to how much weight you can lower, by how much you can raise. This is a delimiting factor. For example, if you can bench press three hundred pounds, you can easily lower three hundred fifty pounds. For the lowering phase of an exercise to be as productive as the raising phase, you must lower more weight. It's possible to use the negative only technique with conventional exercises but special spotting skills are required. It would be easier for you to simply allow more time (approximately four seconds) to lower the weight when each exercise is being performed.

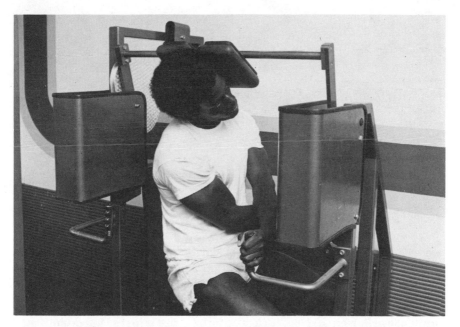

In any exercise, the same muscles are used to raise and lower the weight.

Point: Your muscles will be performing more work, if more time is taken to lower the weight. Because more work is being performed, less weight will be required. The muscles don't know how much weight you're using. Remember that you can de-emphasize the lowering at the expense of raising more weight. A de-emphasis of the lowering phase, however, will be at the expense of maximal results.

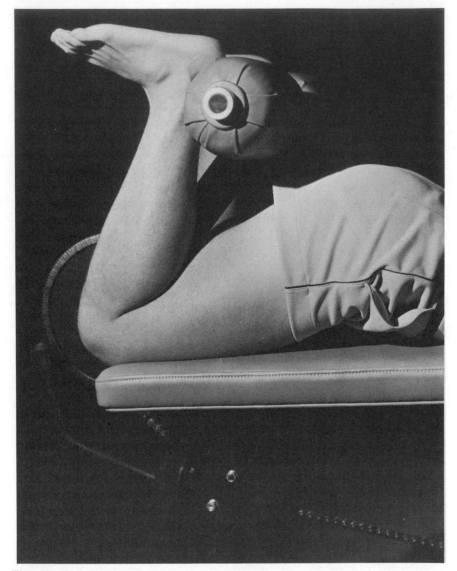

The negative (lowering) phase of a specific exercise is just as important, if not more important, than the positive (raising) phase.

CHECKPOINT #4: OVERLOAD THE MUSCLES PROPERLY

A muscle will gain strength if it is overloaded properly. The overload principle simply states that in order for improvement to occur you must place a demand on the muscle. No demand, no improvement. Less demand than you are capable of handling, less improvement than you are capable of achieving.

Considerable research and pragmatic observations indicate that maximal demand (and therefore maximal results) occur when an exercise is continued for at least forty seconds but not more than seventy seconds to a point of muscular fatigue.

How many repetitions should be performed to achieve maximal demand? The speed of each repetition will dictate how many reps should be performed in a set. If each rep is executed using the methods that have already been described, it should take you at least five to six seconds to complete each repetition of an exercise.

Therefore, you should have time to perform approximately ten to twelve reps. If maximum gains are to be obtained, you must continue exercising until you can no longer perform another repetition correctly. This is called momentary muscular failure. At that point in the exercise, your muscles are temporarily exhausted.

Regardless of the number of reps performed you must reach failure if maximum gains are to be obtained. Why must muscle failure be reached? Common sense tells you that all available muscle fibers have not been used if an exercise is terminated prematurely.

Let's assume that you can properly perform nine reps and will fail on the tenth rep of an exercise but stop at eight reps. You could have performed two more reps but didn't. Those last two reps are the most difficult and most productive reps that can be performed. By not performing those last two reps, you have denied the muscles involved the opportunity to recruit those additional muscle fibers that have not been recruited yet.

Only those fibers that have been recruited will be overloaded. Only those fibers that have been overloaded will get stronger.

Hopefully, the point is clear. **Anything less than an all out effort will produce less than maximum gains.**

Individuals can't measure what constitutes 50%, or 80%, or 99% of a maximum effort. You can only measure what you think is 100% effort. This is obviously a hit-or-miss proposition. The **only** way to measure a 100% effort accurately is to continue an exercise until you can't perform the exercise properly any more.

The same will hold true regardless of the number of sets or reps you do. How do you know when you've reached temporary muscle failure? When you can't raise the weight for another rep.

While performing bench presses, for example, muscular failure is reached when the bar is resting on your chest and you can't raise it off. You've failed while performing the squat, when you're in the squatting position and can't stand up.

Must you exercise to the point of failure to gain strength? No! But to develop maximum gains in strength—yes. Anything short of an all out effort will produce less than maximum gains.

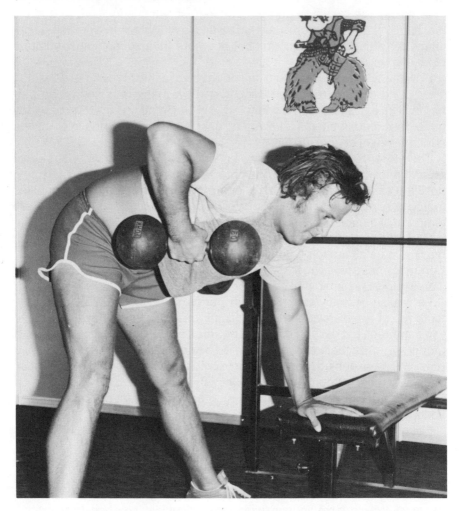

Anything short of an all out effort will produce less than maximum gains.

CHECKPOINT #5: SUPERVISION

The key to maximum gains is supervision. The key to optimum results in any activity is supervision. You should not perform an exercise alone. Without one-on-one supervision, if you are performing an exercise improperly, you will make mistakes unless someone corrects the mistakes.

Is it possible to make good gains without supervision? Sure it is. Anyone can get stronger. You shouldn't accept a level of "just getting stronger." You should commit yourself to a program which will produce maximum gains.

Time may also be a factor. Supervision will help guarantee the best gains in the least amount of time.

What is meant by supervision? Is it one coach, for example, in the weight room with twenty athletes working out on their own?

Proper supervision means one-on-one supervision. Every lifter must have a training partner. Ideally, in an athletic situation, a coach would train each of his/her athletes one on one. In most situations, however, this is impossible—ideal, but impossible.

The next best option for coaches is to assign each athlete a training partner (teammate). Each partner in a training team is responsible for training his/her partner.

The responsibilities of the training partner (spotter) include:

- Prevent injury to the lifter.
- Observe each repetition to insure that the lifter strictly adheres to Checkpoints 1-4.
- Verbally encourage the lifter to help motivate (example: "good job, come on, you can do one more rep, don't quit").
- Verbally discourage the lifter if the exercise is being performed incorrectly (example: "that is not a good rep, you let the weight drop too fast");.

Point: The key to maximum gains is supervision.

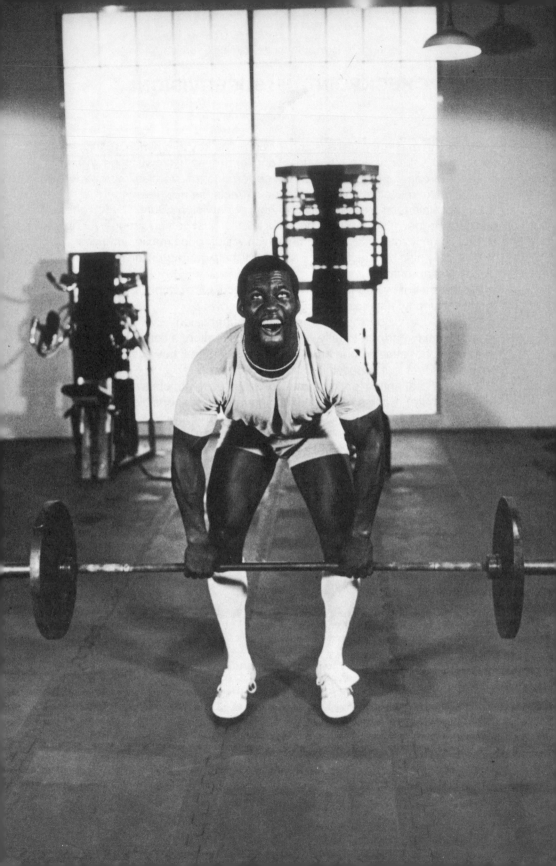

11

FREE WEIGHT EXERCISES

by
James A. Peterson, Ph.D.
Director of Sports Medicine
Women's Sports Foundation

If you have access to free weights, you can implement a selection of the following exercises into your program. The exercises include all the major muscles of your body. Whenever possible, you should perform the exercises in the following order:

1. Dead lift	14. Bent over rowing
2. Parallel squat	15. Bent over flys
3. Good morning	16. Seated press
4. Leg curl with partner	17. Side lateral raise
5. Leg extension with partner	18. Upright row
6. Heel raise	19. Shoulder shrug
7. Foot flexion with partner	20. Bicep curl
8. Bench press	21. French curl
9. Incline press	22. Wrist curl
10. Decline press	23. Reverse wrist curl
11. Bent arm flys	24. Sit-ups
12. Parallel dips	25. Neck series with partner
13. Chin-ups	

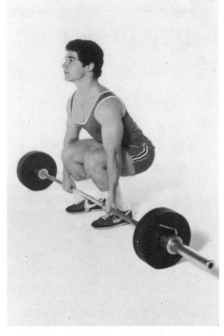 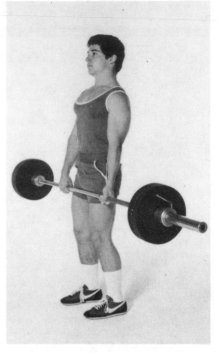

Dead lift: starting position.   **Dead lift: mid-range position.**

DEAD LIFT

Muscles used: Spinal erectors, gluteus maximus, quadriceps

Starting position: Stand with feet slightly greater than shoulder width; squat and grip bar with an underhand grip on non-dominant hand and an overhand grip on dominant hand; keep elbows outside of knees and head up.

Description of the exercise: Pull bar straightening legs and back until standing straight with shoulders back; pause and slowly recover to the starting position and repeat.

Points of significance:
- Keep back straight and lift with legs.
- Keep bar close to shins throughout the exercise.
- Roll shoulders back at completion of positive movement.

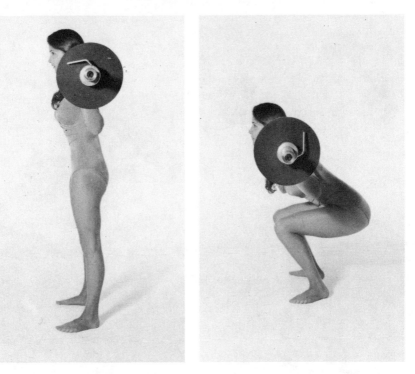

Parallel squat: starting position.   **Parallel squat: mid-range position.**

PARALLEL SQUAT

Muscles used: Buttocks, quadriceps

Starting position: Stand with your feet approximately shoulder width apart, barbell resting on your trapezius and posterior deltoids.

Description of the exercise: Lower the buttocks until your thighs are at least parallel to the floor, pause momentarily and recover to the starting position.

Spotting: The spotter should stand behind you as close as possible without interfering with the lift. If you need assistance in recovering to the starting position, the spotter should place his/her arms around your chest and pull up until you are in the upright position. This will prevent you from folding at the waist and possibly injuring your lower back.

Points to emphasize:
- Look upward when performing the exercise.
- Try to keep the bar in line with the base of support (the feet).
- Eliminate any bouncing during the squatting portion of the exercise (such bouncing can damage the knee joint).

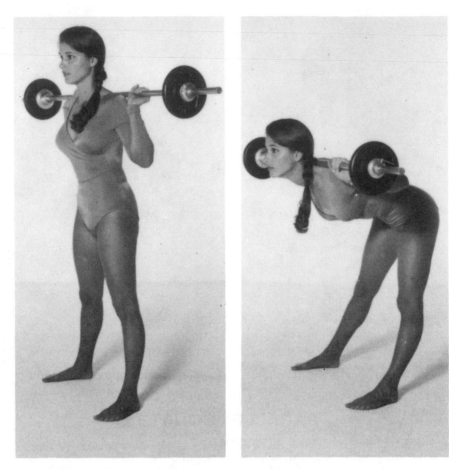

Good morning: starting position.　　**Good morning: mid-range position.**

GOOD MORNING

Muscles used: Lower back

Starting position: Stand with the barbell behind your neck resting on your shoulders; your feet should be spread shoulder width apart; your legs locked.

Description of the exercise: Bend forward at the waist until your body is below parallel with the floor; pause momentarily and recover to the starting position.

Points of significance: Keep your head up throughout the exercise.

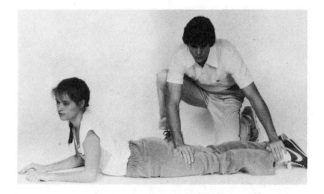

Leg curl: starting position.

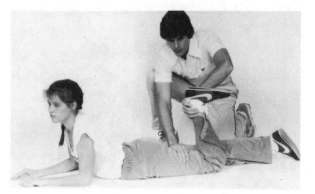

Leg curl: mid-range position.

LEG CURL

Muscles used: Hamstrings

Starting position: Lie flat on ground with both legs extended; partner places hands behind your left heel.

Description of the exercise: While your partner applies resistance, curl your foot as high as possible (at least perpendicular); pause, slowly recover to starting position and repeat. When your left leg is exhausted, perform same exercise with your right leg.

Points of significance:

- Your partner should apply enough resistance so that a maximum effort takes approximately two seconds for the positive movement and four seconds for the negative.
- Keep your body flat on the ground.

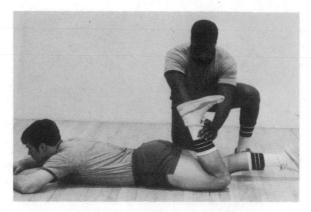

Leg extension: starting position.

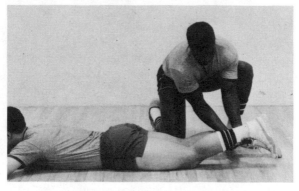

Leg extension: mid-range position.

LEG EXTENSION

Muscles used: Quadriceps

Starting position: Lie flat on ground with your left leg flexed as far as possible. Your partner places his/her hands in front of your left foot.

Description of the exercise: While your partner applies resistance, push your foot back and downward until your leg is extended; pause and slowly recover to the starting position and repeat. When your left leg is exhausted, perform same exercise with your right leg.

Points of significance:

- Your partner should apply enough resistance so that a maximum effort takes two seconds for the positive movement and four seconds for the negative.
- Do not raise your knee off the ground.

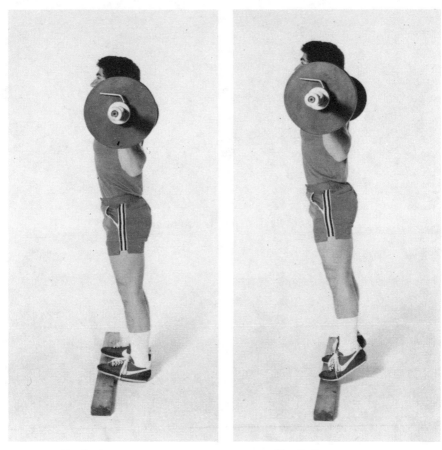

Heel raise:
starting position.

Heel raise:
mid-range position.

HEEL RAISE

Muscles used: Calves

Starting position: Stand with a barbell across your shoulders; your toes should be elevated to provide maximum stretching.

Description of the exercise: Raise your heels off the floor, while rising up on your toes; pause and slowly recover to the starting position.

Points of significance:
- Elevate your heels as high as possible each repetition.
- Raise your heels slowly.
- Emphasize the lowering phase of the exercise.

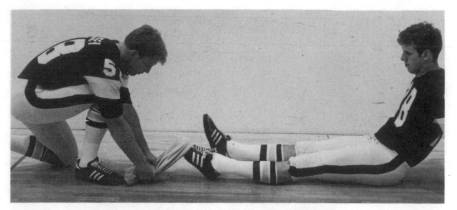

Foot flexion: mid-range position.

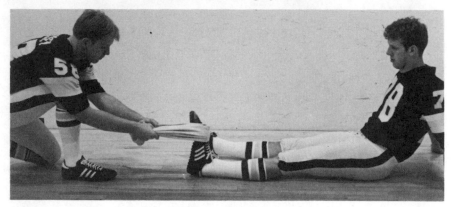

Foot flexion: starting position.

FOOT FLEXION

Muscles used: Tibialis anterior

Starting position: Sit on ground with both legs extended and feet flexed; your partner loops towel over toes on right foot.

Description of the exercise: Your partner applies enough resistance so that a maximum effort takes two seconds for the positive movement and four seconds for the negative phase; pause and slowly recover to the starting position and repeat. When your right leg is exhausted, repeat exercise with your left leg.

Points of significance:

- Place the towel high on your toes for maximum leverage.
- Keep your knee straight throughout the movement.

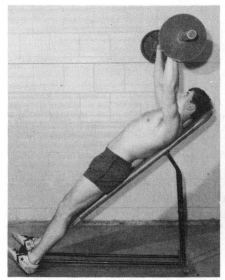

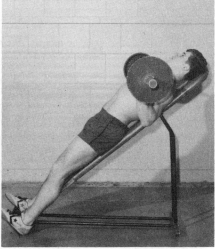

Incline press: mid-range position.

Incline press: starting position.

INCLINE PRESS

Muscles used: Pectorals, deltoids, triceps

Starting position: Lie on your back on an incline bench with a barbell or dumbbells in the arms-extended position.

Description of the exercise: Lower the weight to the top of your rib cage and recover to the arms-extended position.

Spotting: The spotter should stand to the rear of you giving assistance when needed by placing his/her hands on your wrist. This allows the spotter to assist you in maintaining control of the bar or dumbbell.

Points of significance:

- Dumbbells (if used) should be held so that your palms are facing away from your body.
- As you fatigue, the tendency will be for the dumbbells to fall away from the center of your body; therefore, when extending your arms, you should bring the dumbbells together in the arms-extended position.
- Lower the bar so that it remains perpendicular to the floor (not to your body).

BENCH PRESS

Muscles used: Pectorals, deltoids, triceps

Starting position: Lie face up on an exercise bench with your knees bent and your feet flat on the floor; your buttocks and shoulder blades should be in contact with the bench; the barbell is in the arms-extended position.

Description of the exercise: Lower the barbell to your chest; pause momentarily and recover to the starting position.

Spotting: The spotter should assist you into the starting position. If you are unable to complete a repetition, the spotter should assist you only as much as is needed to complete the repetition. You will need assistance when the bar is nearest your chest. The spotter should bend at the waist with his/her hands under the bar and not over it.

Points of significance:

- Do not arch your back. This could provide a mechanical advantage but may cause injury to the lower back.
- You should lower the bar to your chest each repetition and touch your chest at the same spot without bouncing the bar; you should maintain eye contact with the bar throughout the exercise.
- With your arms vertical to the floor, the barbell should be lowered to your chest in a straight line.
- When recovering to the starting position, the barbell should be pressed upward and slightly backward so that upon completion of the repetition, the barbell is approximately over the neck (a readjustment to the vertical position is necessary before initiating the next repetition).
- Dumbbells may be used to perform this exercise.

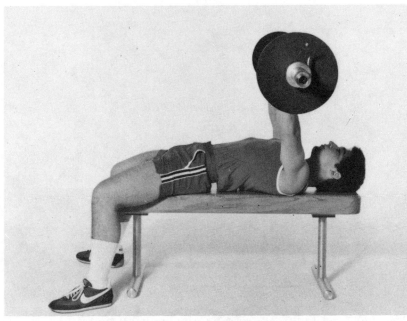

Bench press: starting position.

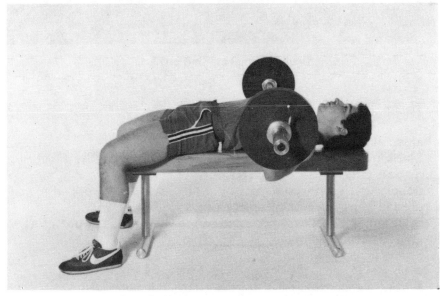

Bench press: mid-range position.

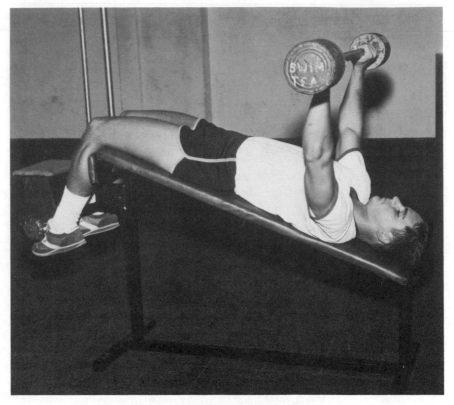

Decline press: starting position.

DECLINE PRESS

Muscles used: Pectorals, deltoids, triceps

Starting position: Lie on your back on a decline bench with the barbell or dumbbells in the arms-extended position.

Description of the exercise: Lower the bar to the lower part of your chest and then recover to the arms-extended position.

Spotting: The spotter should stand behind you and assist you by placing his/her hands on your wrist.

Points of significance:

- Lower the bar so that it remains perpendicular to the floor.
- Bring dumbbells together in the arms extended position.
- Lower the dumbbells simultaneously.

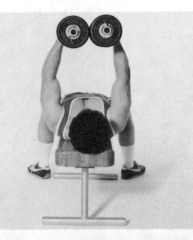

Bent arm flys: starting position.

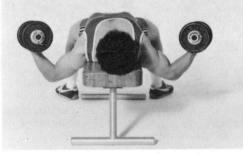

Bent arm flys: mid-range position.

BENT ARM FLYS

Muscles used: Pectorals

Starting position: Lie on your back on a bench with your arms extended in a semi-flexed position.

Description of the exercise: Lower the dumbbells downward and sideward while maintaining the semi-flexed position of your arms; then recover to the starting position.

Points of significance:
- Keep your arms locked in a semi-flexed position.
- Allow your pectorals to be stretched maximally when the weight is being lowered.
- Raise and lower your arms as if hugging a barrel.

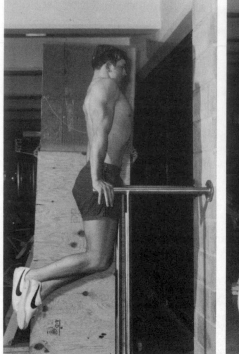 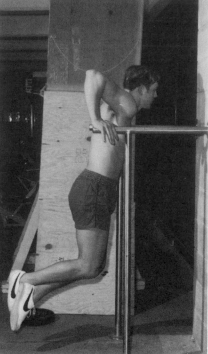

Parallel dips:
starting position.

Parallel dips:
mid-range position.

PARALLEL DIPS

Muscles used: Pectorals, deltoids, triceps

Starting position: Mount the dip bars with your arms extended; grip the bars with your hands facing inward; suspend your weight with your elbows slightly bent and your knees bent.

Description of the exercise: Slowly lower your body as far as possible; pause and recover to the starting position.

Points of significance:

- Bend your knees so that a full range of movement can be obtained while lowering your body.
- Additional weight should be added to your body once you can perform 12 properly executed repetitions.
- Lower your body slowly (4 seconds).
- This exercise can be performed in negative-only fashion. A stool or steps will be needed to raise your body.

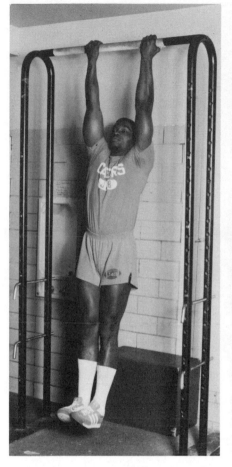 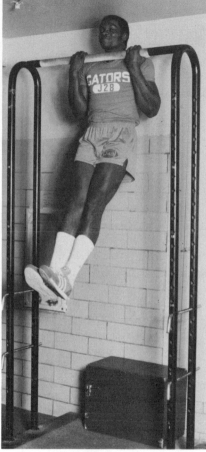

Chin ups:
starting position.

Chin ups:
mid-range position.

CHIN UPS

Muscles used: Latissimus dorsi, biceps

Starting position: Grip the bar with an underhand grip and with your hands shoulder width apart; hang from the bar with your elbows straight.

Description of the exercise: Raise your body upward until your chin is above the bar; pause and slowly recover to the starting position.

Points of significance:

- Do not allow your body to swing during the exercise.
- Allow your elbows to extend completely at bottom of the movement.

145

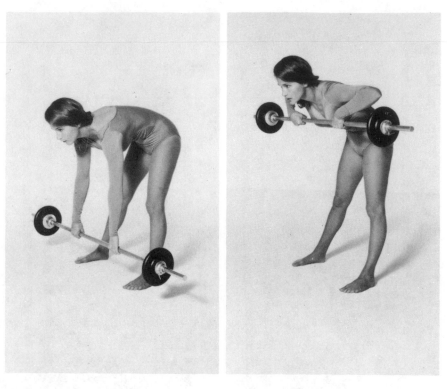

Bent over rowing: starting position.   **Bent over rowing: mid-range position.**

BENT OVER ROWING

Muscles used: Latissimus dorsi, biceps

Starting position: Stand with your body bent forward at the waist so that your upper body is parallel to the floor, feet shoulder width apart, knees slightly flexed (to take the pressure off your lower back).

Description of the exercise: Pull the barbell upward so that the barbell touches your chest; pause momentarily and recover to the starting position.

Points of significance:

- A bench may be used to rest your forehead upon in order to stabilize your body in the bent over position.
- Keep the back of your hand on top of the bar; do not flex your wrists.
- Do not pull the weight toward your stomach. The bar should travel in a line that is perpendicular to the floor.
- An inefficient exercise for the lats, the biceps will fail first; when this occurs, you will not be able to pull the bar all the way up to your chest.

146

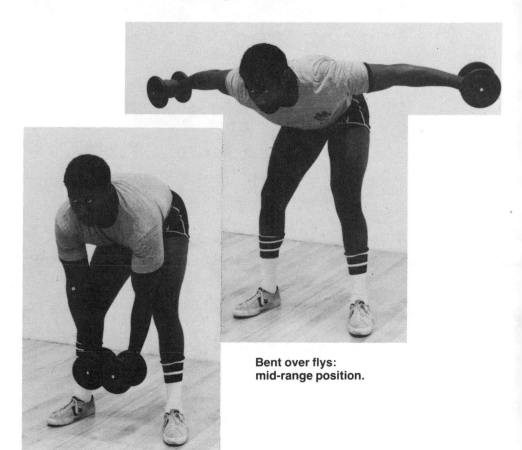

**Bent over flys:
mid-range position.**

**Bent over flys:
starting position.**

BENT OVER FLYS

Muscles used: Latissimus dorsi, rhomboids

Starting position: Stand with your feet shoulder width apart and your knees slightly bent; bend forward at waist until your torso is parallel with floor; grip dumbbells with palms facing inward, arms straight, and dumbbells touching each other.

Description of exercise: Raise your arms laterally as high as possible; pause and slowly recover to the starting position.

Points of significance:

- Keep your head up and your back straight.
- Keep your back parallel to floor throughout the exercise.

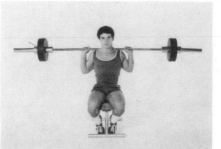

Seated press: starting position.

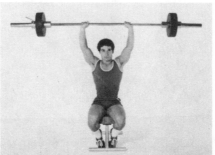

Seated press: mid-range position.

SEATED PRESS

Muscles used: Deltoids, triceps

Starting position: Sit on an exercise bench with the barbell resting on your shoulders behind your neck; your feet should be hooked on the bench legs to prevent you from falling backwards.

Description of the exercise: Raise the weight so that your arms become momentarily extended; recover to the starting position.

Spotting: The spotter should stand behind you to assist you in raising the weight if necessary.

Points of significance:

- Lower the barbell completely so that it touches the base of your neck (each repetition).
- Do not lean back when extending your arms; this is a form of cheating. The weight you are using is probably too heavy and you are trying to recruit the pectorals to assist. It also places undue stress on your lower back.
- Dumbbells may be used. If dumbbells are used, it is suggested that they be raised and lowered alternately.

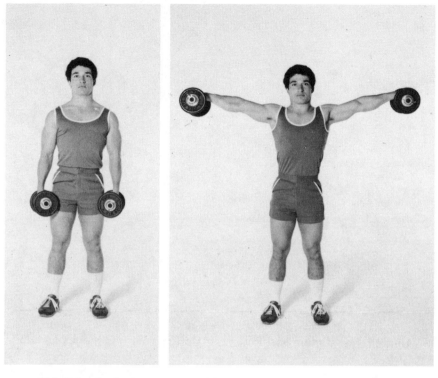

Side lateral raise: starting position.

Side lateral raise: mid-range position.

SIDE LATERAL RAISE

Muscles used: Deltoids

Starting position: Stand with your arms extended downward; palms facing each other with the dumbbells touching in front of your body; your body should be slightly bent forward at the waist.

Description of the exercise: Raise the dumbbells sideward and upward so that the dumbbells are approximately parallel with your head; pause momentarily and recover to the starting position.

Spotting: A spotter can apply resistance (manually) to your hands while you raise your arms sideward and upward (this will eliminate the need for using dumbbells).

Points of significance:
- Stand as straight as possible.
- Do not raise the weights above the level of your shoulders, otherwise other muscles will become involved.

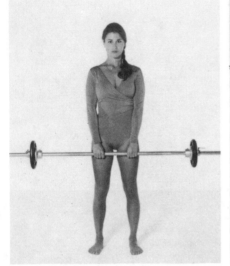 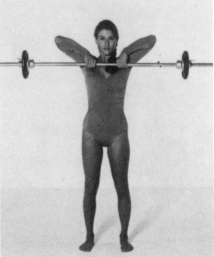

Upright row: starting position.   **Upright row: mid-range position.**

UPRIGHT ROW

Muscles used: Deltoids, biceps, trapezius

Starting position: Stand with your arms extended downward with the barbell in both hands; a closer than shoulder width grip should be used; your feet should be shoulder width apart.

Description of the exercise: Pull the barbell upward and touch your chin with the bar; pause momentarily and recover to the starting position.

Points of significance:
- Do not bend at the waist (stand perfectly straight).
- Raise and lower the bar all the way to your chin in a straight line.
- Let your shoulder girdle relax when your arms are completely extended.

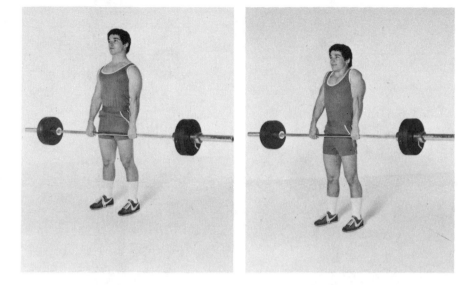

Shoulder shrug:
starting position.

Shoulder shrug:
mid-range position.

SHOULDER SHRUG

Muscles used: Trapezius

Starting position: Stand with your feet shoulder width apart and your arms extended downward; grip bar with an overhand grip; your hands should be shoulder width apart.

Description of the exercise: Keep your arms straight and raise your shoulders as high as possible; pause and slowly recover to the starting position.

Points of significance:

- Stand straight throughout exercise.
- Allow your shoulders to drop as far as possible at bottom of movement.
- Do not bend your arms when raising the weight.

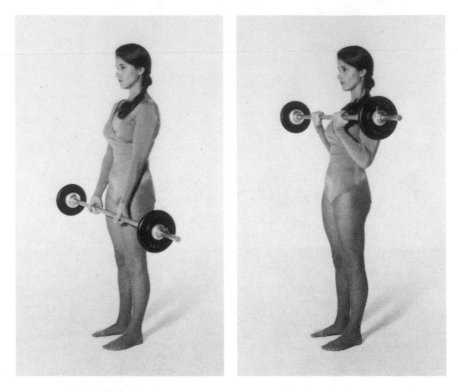

**Biceps curl:
starting position.**

**Biceps curl:
mid-range position.**

BICEPS CURL

Muscles used: Biceps

Starting position: Stand with your feet less than shoulder width apart and your arms extended downward; grip the bar with an underhand grip, your hands just outside of your hips.

Description of exercise: Keep your elbows back and curl the bar as high as possible; pause and slowly recover to the starting position.

Points of significance:

- Keep your back straight and do not lean back.
- Keep your elbows back throughout exercise.
- Lower the weight slowly.
- If dumbbells are used, you should alternate raising and lowering the weight.
- If dumbbells are used, one dumbbell should always be held in the contracted position.

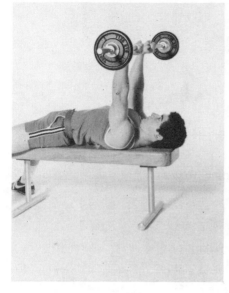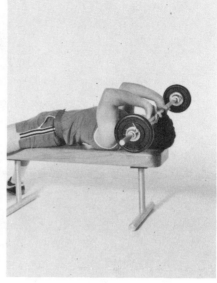

French curl: starting position.   **French curl: mid-range position.**

FRENCH CURL

Muscles used: Triceps

Starting position: Lie on your back on an exercise bench with your feet flat on the floor; the barbell should be in the arms-extended position with your arms vertical to the floor; grip the bar with an overhand grip, with your hands held narrower than shoulder width.

Description of the exercise: Bending only at the elbow, lower the barbell to your forehead and recover to the starting position.

Spotting: The spotter should hand you the barbell to assist you into the starting position. Upon completion of the exercise, the spotter should replace the barbell to the floor.

Points of significance:

- Your upper arms should remain vertical to the floor throughout the exercise.
- Keep your elbows at shoulder width throughout the exercise.
- The exercise may be performed while in a seated position; however, it is very difficult to keep your elbows in and your upper arms perpendicular to the floor in this position.

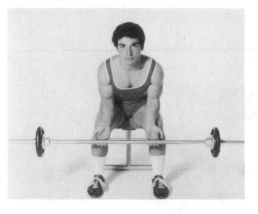

Wrist curl: starting position.

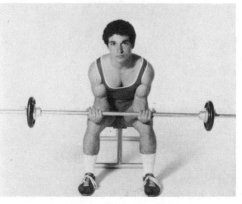

Wrist curl: mid-range position.

WRIST CURL

Muscles used: Forearm flexors

Starting position: Sit on end of bench with your knees bent and your feet flat on floor; place your forearms firmly against your thighs; grip the bar with an underhand grip and allow the bar to roll to your finger tips.

Description of the exercise: Curl your fingers upward and flex your wrists; pause and slowly recover to the starting position.

Points of significance:

- Keep your forearms in contact with your thighs throughout the exercise.
- Allow your fingers to extend downward as far as possible at bottom of the movement.

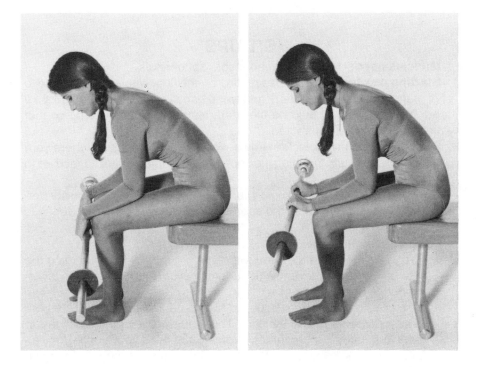

Reverse wrist curl: starting position.   Reverse wrist curl: mid-range position.

REVERSE WRIST CURL

Muscles used: Forearm extensors

Starting position: Sit on end of a bench with your knees bent and your feet flat on floor; place your forearms firmly against your thighs; grip the bar with an overhand grip and allow your wrists to bend downward.

Description of the exercise: Curl your wrists upward and backward as far as possible; pause and slowly recover to starting position.

Points of significance:
- Keep your forearms in contact with your thighs throughout the exercise.
- Keep your wrists just over the ends of your knees.

SIT UPS

Muscles used: Hip flexors, quadriceps, abdominals

Starting position: Sit on a pad resting on the floor with your feet close to your buttocks, knees together, and your hands interlocked behind your head. Your buttocks should be elevated; lean slightly backwards so that your abdominals are contracted.

Description of the exercise: Lower your body to a position where your upper back is not quite touching the floor; pause momentarily and recover to the starting position.

Spotting: A spotter should hold your feet if necessary. When you are performing negative only situps, the spotter should assist you in recovering to the starting position.

Points of significance:

- Your hips should be elevated to prevent your back from touching the floor; this will help prevent your abdominals from momentarily recovering during each repetition.
- When raising your upper body, do not come to a position where your torso is perpendicular to the floor. This would allow your abdominals to relax and recover momentarily. You should raise your upper body as far as possible as long as you can maintain tension on your abdominals.
- Allow your muscles to raise your body, not by momentum. Raise the body slowly while keeping the elbows stationary. It should take approximately 2 seconds to raise your body.
- It should take approximately 3-4 seconds to lower your body.
- The demand can be increased by placing a barbell plate on the chest. It should not be held behind your head since this would place more stress on your lower back. A spotter may also provide additional resistance by pulling you downward while you lower your torso.
- The higher your hips are elevated, the greater the difficulty and the greater the stress on your lower back. Be cautious. You should adapt to the elevation of your hips slowly and support your lower back if necessary.

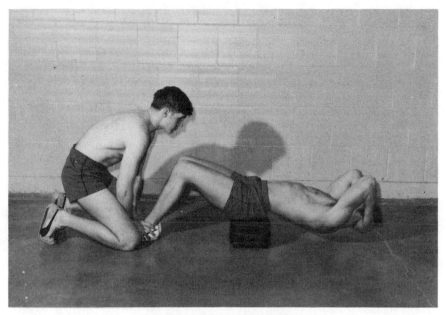

Situps: starting position.

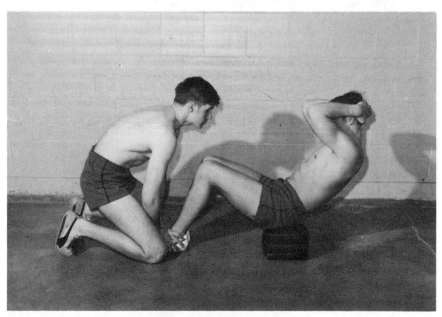

Situps: mid-range position.

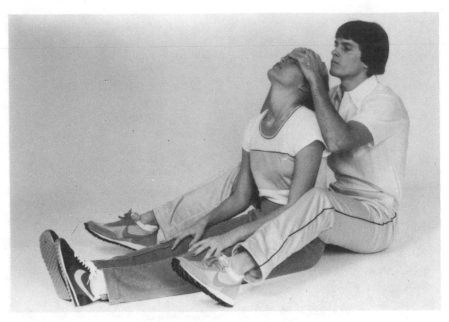

Neck flexion: starting position.

NECK FLEXION

Muscles used: Neck flexors

Starting position: Sit with your back and hands resting against your partner. Your neck at the beginning of each repetition should be totally relaxed and you should look upward.

Description of exercise: Lower your head downward (taking 4 seconds) until your chin touches your chest; recover to the starting position without any resistance from your partner.

Spotter: Your partner clasps his/her hands over your forehead and places a mild pre-stretch on your neck. As you lower your head, your partner should decrease the pressure accordingly. When a repetition is completed, your partner releases his/her hands and allows you to recover to the starting position without applying any resistance.

Points of significance:
- Take approximately four seconds to complete each repetition.
- Do not jerk your head. All movements should be controlled, smooth, and slow.
- Perform approximately 10 repetitions of the exercise.

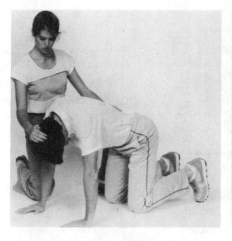
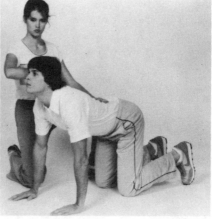

Neck extension: starting position. **Neck extension: mid-range position.**

NECK EXTENSION

Muscles used: Neck extensors

Starting position: Assume an all-fours position with your neck totally relaxed and your chin touching your chest.

Description of exercise: Lift your head upward and backward until your neck is fully extended and hold this position momentarily. Take approximately 4 seconds to complete each repetition.

Spotting: Your partner places his/her hand on the back of your head and gently applies pressure to stretch the neck muscles. As you raise your head, your partner should apply direct pressure to your head and vary the resistance throughout the exercise; recover to the starting position without any resistance being applied by your partner.

Points of significance:

- Take approximately 4 seconds to complete each repetition.
- Do not jerk your head. All movements should be controlled, smooth, and slow.
- Perform approximately 10 repetitions of the exercise.

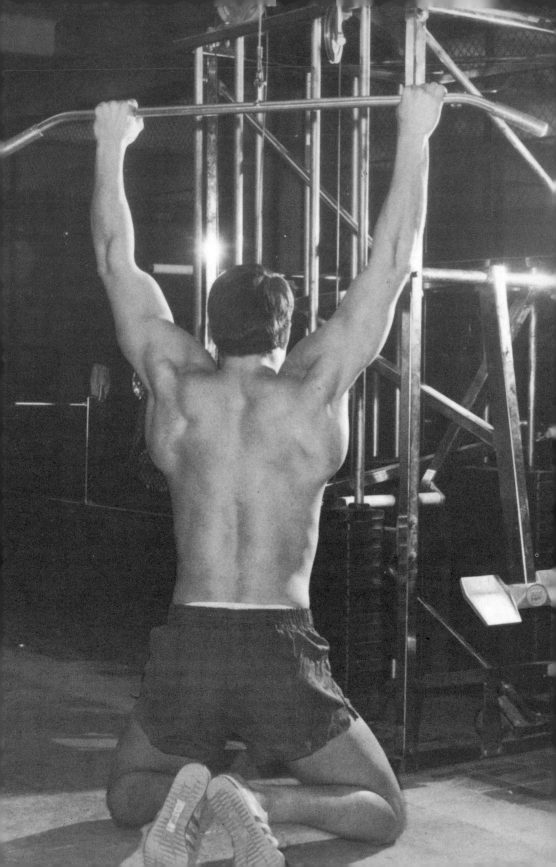

12

UNIVERSAL GYM EXERCISES

by
Joe Diange
Penn State University

If you have access to Universal Gym Equipment, you can implement the following exercises into your program. The exercises involve all the major muscles of your body. Whenever possible, you should perform the exercises in the order listed:

1. Leg press	9. Back extension
2. Leg extension	10. Dips
3. Leg curl	11. Lat pulldown
4. Bench press	12. L-Seat dips
5. Chinup	13. Biceps curls
6. Side lateral raise	14. Neck flexion
7. Seated press	15. Neck extension
8. Upright rows	16. Shrugs

LEG PRESS

Muscles used: Major muscles of the legs, buttocks.

Starting position: Sit with the middle of your feet on the leg press pedals. If both upper and lower foot pedals are available, use the upper pedals. The seat should be adjusted so that your upper and lower leg form an angle of less than 90°; place your hands on the side of the seat to hold your buttocks down.

Description: Extend your legs to a position just before "locking them out." Do not extend your legs completely (this will allow the muscles to recover momentarily). Recover to the starting position without letting the weight plates lifted touch the weight plates which are not lifted.

Spotting: The spotter should place one foot on the leg pedals on the first rep to help you start the exercise. If you fail before performing the prescribed number of reps (12), the spotter can help you raise the weight by pushing on the foot pedal with his foot. Keep in mind that you will be capable of lowering the weight without assistance. If the weight is too light, the spotter can apply additional pressure to the weight stack forcing you to fail by the 12th repetition.

Points to emphasize:

- If you should get a headache, relax your shoulders and neck and move the seat back.
- If a separate leg extension and leg curl station is available, the leg extension exercise should be performed first and the leg press second.

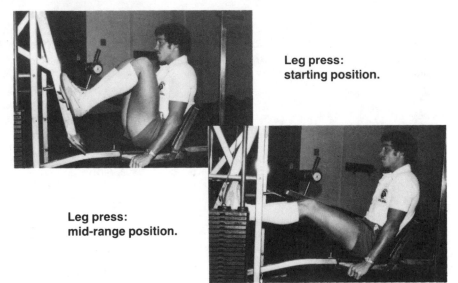

Leg press:
starting position.

Leg press:
mid-range position.

162

LEG EXTENSION

Muscles used: Quadriceps.

Starting position: Sit on the leg extension machine, leaning back slightly with your hands grasping the sides of the machine.

Description: Extend your legs forward and upward; **pause momentarily** in the extended position, recover to the starting position.

Points to emphasize:

- Do not count the rep if you cannot pause in the contracted position.
- Reach the extended position each rep.
- Keep your buttocks on the seat at all times; don't lean forward.
- Additional padding can be placed on the rollers for both comfort and greater prestretching of the muscle.

Leg extension: starting position.

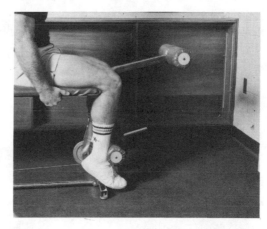

Leg extension: mid-range position.

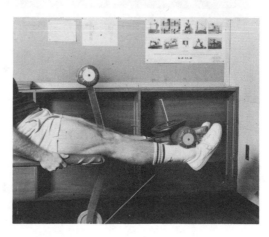

LEG CURL

Muscles used: Hamstrings.

Starting position: Lie face down on the leg curl machine with your heels hooked under the pads or rollers; your kneecaps should be just off the edge of the pad for maximum comfort. Your toes should remain pointed toward the knees throughout the performance of the exercise.

Description: Flex your lower legs raising them forward and upward as far as possible; **pause momentarily** in the contracted position, then recover to the starting position..

Spotting: If you fail before the 12th rep, the spotter can help you raise the weight to the mid-range position.

Points to emphasize:
- Raise the weight so that your lower legs are at least perpendicular to the floor.
- Wrap additional padding on the rollers to provide for additional stretching in the starting position.

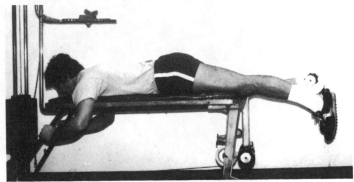

Leg curl: starting position.

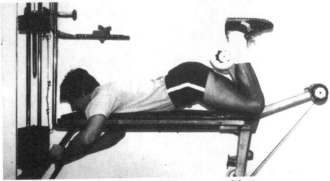

Leg curl: mid-range position.

BENCH PRESS

Muscles used: Chest, shoulders, triceps.

Starting position: Lie on a bench with your knees bent and your feet flat on the floor. The bench press handles should bisect the middle of your chest. The bench should be elevated to place the chest muscles in a stretched position when the weight is lowered. Your arms should be extended.

Description: Lower the bar to the mid-range position. Then recover to the starting position and repeat. The weight plates which are lifted should not touch the remainder of the weight stack in the mid-range position.

Spotting: The spotter should help you raise the weight so that you can begin the exercise in the arms-extended position.

Points to emphasize:

- Blocks of wood of different sizes can be used to vary the height of the bench. The thickness of your rib cage will determine how high the bench should be raised. If the bench is too low, you will not achieve full range exercise.

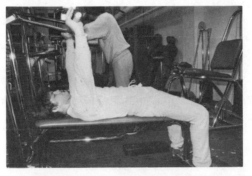

Bench press: starting position.

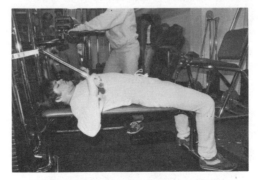

Bench press: mid-range position.

CHINUPS

Muscles used: Lats, biceps.

Starting position: Hang from a chinup bar using an underhand (palms towards your face) closer than shoulder-width grip.

Description: Pull your body upward so that your chin is over (not resting on) the bar; pause momentarily, recover to the starting position.

Spotting: If, and when, you perform negative-only chins, the spotter should add additional resistance by pulling on your hips while you lower your body weight.

Points to emphasize:
- A bar should be welded to the chin station to form one solid chin bar. This will allow you to take a proper width grip when performing the chinup.
- A weight belt will be needed to add additional weight to the athlete who can properly perform 10-12 reps with his own body weight. If such a belt is not available, a spotter can pull down on the lifter's hips to add extra resistance.
- Steps or a ladder will be needed if you cannot properly perform 10-12 reps. This will allow you to continue performing chinups in negative-only fashion.
- The attachment point of the chin bar to the Universal machine can be used as the chinup station. It is closer to the floor which will eliminate your climbing to the much higher conventional station. This will also make negative-only chins easier and safer to perform. Pad the attachment point to prevent possible injury to your chin. You must bend your legs to prevent them from touching the floor.

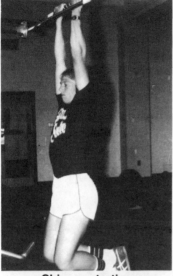

Chinup: starting position.

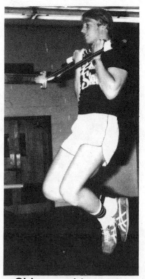

Chinup: mid-range position.

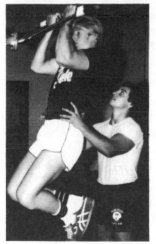

A spotter can add additional weight by pulling on your hips.

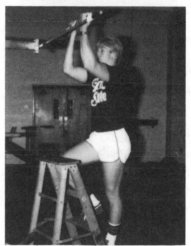

You can use steps or a ladder to raise your body when performing negative-only chinups.

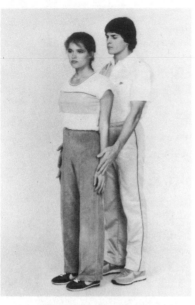

Side lateral raise:
starting position.

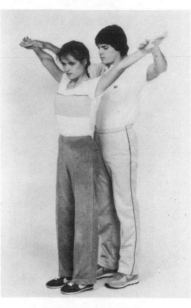

Side lateral raise:
mid-range position.

SIDE LATERAL RAISE

Muscles used: Deltoids

Starting position: Stand upright with your arms hanging down but not touching your sides.

Description of exercise: Raise your arms sideward and upward until they are slightly more than parallel to the floor, pause momentarily, recover to the starting position.

Spotting: Your partner, standing behind you, places his/her hands on your wrists and manually applies pressure on them throughout the exercise. Keep in mind that you can lower more than you can raise; therefore, your partner must apply greater pressure during the lowering phase.

Points of significance:

- Keep tension on your muscles throughout the exercise.
- The movement of your arms should be smooth and steady throughout the exercise.
- The first few reps should be done at a sub-maximum effort. Thereafter, you should exert an all-out effort. If performed correctly, you should have difficulty raising your arms the last few reps.
- Because you are tiring each succeeding rep, your partner should vary and decrease the resistance accordingly.

SEATED PRESS

Muscles used: Shoulders, chest, triceps.

Starting position: Sit on a stool and face away from the machine. Your legs should be bent and your feet elevated off the floor (to help keep your lower back flat). Your lower back should be kept flat throughout the exercise. The higher your feet are elevated the flatter your back will remain.

Description: Raise the weight, extending your arms completely; recover to the starting position.

Points to emphasize:

- Do not arch your back in an attempt to raise the weight. Arching the back will place considerable stress on your back.
- In the arms-extended position, the bar should be directly over your shoulders.
- In the starting position, the handle base should be just behind your shoulders.

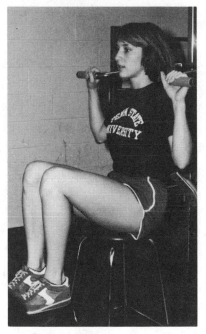

**Seated press:
starting position.
The feet are elevated
to keep the lower back flat.**

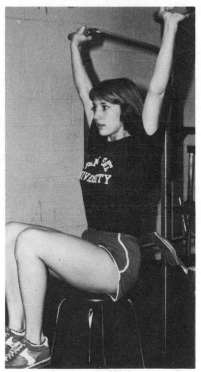

**Seated press:
mid-range position.**

UPRIGHT ROWS

Muscles used: Deltoids, trapezius, biceps.

Starting position: Stand holding a barbell in an arms-extended downward position; grip the bar with a closer than shoulder width grip; your feet should be shoulder width apart; your head looking skyward.

Description: Pull the bar upward touching the bar under your chin; **pause** momentarily, recover to the starting position.

Spotting: If you fail before the 12th rep, the spotter should help you raise the weight; if it is too light, the spotter should apply additional resistance for the remaining reps.

Points to emphasize:

- This exercise can be performed using either a Universal biceps curl station or a barbell. If the Universal biceps curl is used to perform the upright row, a barbell should be used to perform the biceps curl. This will eliminate any backup that may occur if two different exercises are performed at the Universal biceps curl station.
- Do not bend forward at the waist (stand perfectly straight).
- Allow your shoulder girdle to relax totally when your arms are completely extended.

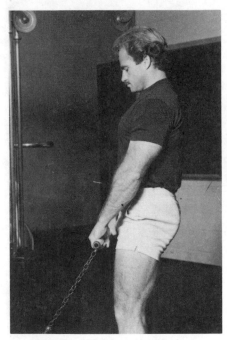

Upright row: starting position.

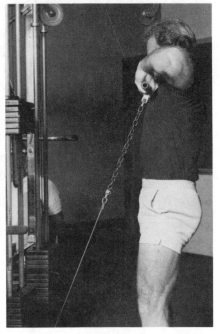

Upright row: mid-range position.

170

BACK EXTENSION

Starting position: Lie face down with your hips resting on a pad so that your upper body is hanging over the bench; your upper body should be perpendicular to the floor; your arms should be folded and held against your chest.

Description: Raise your body forward and upward until your body is parallel to the floor; **pause momentarily**, recover to the starting position.

Spotting: The spotter should place his hands on your upper back and manually apply and vary the resistance throughout the entire exercise. The spotter must insure that you do not raise your body (arch the back) above a point parallel to the floor.

Points to emphasize:

- While stressing your lower back, do not exercise to the point of failure during the first few workouts. Gradually increase the intensity each succeeding workout.
- Do not arch your back. Arching your back can result in an injury to your lower back.
- The spotter must learn to vary the resistance while you raise and lower your body. You are stronger during the lowering of the body than you are during the raising phase of the exercise. For maximum efficiency, the spotter must vary the resistance accordingly. This method of spotting is far superior to placing a weight behind the head.

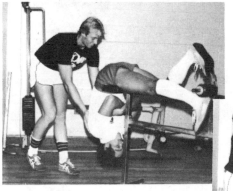

Back extension: starting position.

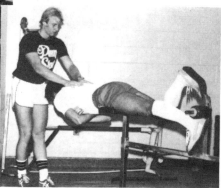

Back extension: mid-range position.

DIPS

Muscles used: Chest, shoulders, triceps.

Starting position: Mount the dip bars with your arms extended and your legs bent (to provide full range during the lowering of your body).

Description: Bend your arms and lower your body as much as possible; pause momentarily; recover to the starting position.

Spotting: The spotter may have to pull on your hips to add additional resistance if you are capable of performing more than 12 reps with your own body weight.

Points to emphasize:

- A weight belt can be used to add additional weight to the athlete who can properly perform 10-12 reps with his own body weight.
- Negative-only dips can be performed if you fail before performing 12 properly executed reps. Steps can be placed at the bottom of the dip station or you can use the back of the leg press seat to step up on to allow you to recover to the starting position.

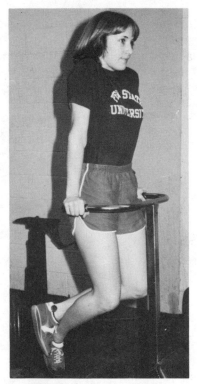

Dips: starting position.

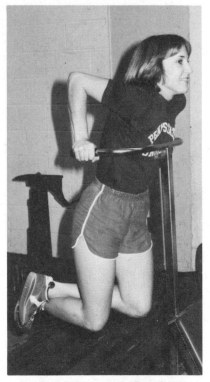

Dips: mid-range position.

LAT PULLDOWN

Muscles used: Latissimus dorsi, biceps, posterior deltoid.

Starting position: Assume a kneeling or seated position on the floor so that the back of your neck is directly under the bar on the lat machine. The weight plates which are being lifted should not touch that part of the weight stack not being lifted. This will provide a prestretch in the starting position.

Description: Pull the bar downward to the base of your neck; **pause momentarily**; recover to the starting position.

Spotting: A spotter may be needed to apply pressure to your shoulders to prevent you from raising off the floor. The spotter can apply pressure to your elbows throughout the entire exercise to allow your lats to do more work and your biceps less work. If this method is used, you will need less weight.

Points to emphasize:

- The lat pulldown bar should be taped to provide a safer grip (chalk or resin can be available). The spotter should be alert to avoid injury to himself should your grip slip and allow the bar to dangerously move upward.
- You should lean forward slightly and **keep your body in that position.**
- Do not use a wide grip. The range of movement is greater for the lats when a moderate grip is used.

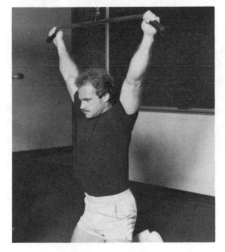 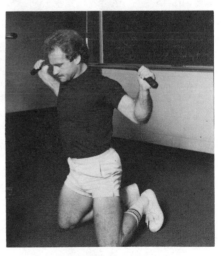

Lat pulldown:
starting position.

Lat pulldown:
mid-range position.

BICEP CURLS

Muscles used: Biceps.

Starting position: In a standing position with your arms fully extended, grasp the curl bar pulley.

Description: Raise the pulley forward and upward to fully contract your biceps while keeping your elbows back slightly; pause momentarily, then recover to the starting position.

Spotting: If a barbell is used, the spotter should manually pull on the bar as the bar is raised and lowered to make the exercise more efficient.

Points to emphasize:

- Do not allow your elbows to come forward or let your upper arms become perpendicular to the floor. This will allow the biceps to rest momentarily unless a spotter is pulling back on the pulley in that position.
- If you perform upright rows on the bicep curl station of the Universal gym, use a barbell to execute the bicep curl. This will prevent two different exercises from being performed on the same station.

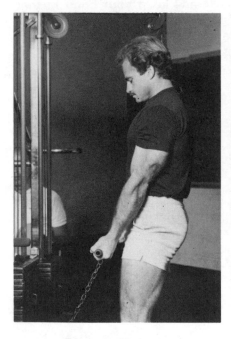

Bicep curls: starting position.

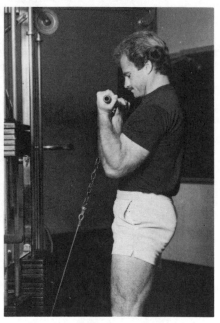

Bicep curls: mid-range position.

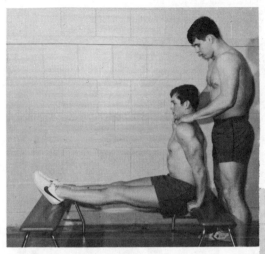

L-seat dips: starting position.

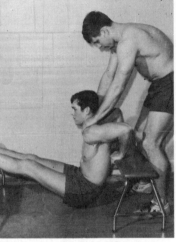

L-seat dips: mid-range position.

L-SEAT DIPS

Muscles used: Triceps, deltoids

Starting position: Position your body either between two benches or on one bench if you want to decrease the difficulty of the exercise; grasp the side of the bench with your hands approximately shoulder width apart.

Description of exercise: Bend your arms and lower your body as far as possible; recover to the starting position.

Spotting: Your partner should stand on the bench and apply as much pressure as needed to cause muscular failure between 8-12 reps.

Points of significance:

- If you reach muscular failure before performing 8 reps, you may bend your legs which will make the exercise easier.

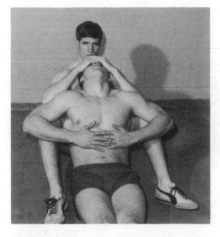

Neck flexion: starting position.

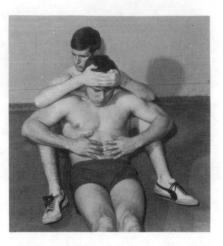

Neck flexion: mid-range position.

NECK FLEXION

Muscles used: Neck flexors

Starting position: Sit with your back and hands resting against your partner. Your neck at the beginning of each repetition should be totally relaxed and looking upward.

Description of exercise: Lower your head downward (taking 4 seconds) until your chin touches your chest; recover to the starting position without any resistance from your partner.

Spotter: Your partner clasps his/her hands over your forehead and places a mild pre-stretch on your neck. As you lower your head, your partner should decrease the pressure accordingly. When a repetition is completed, your partner releases his/her hands and allows you to recover to the starting position without applying any resistance.

Points of significance:

- Take approximately four seconds to complete each repetition.
- Do not jerk your head. All movements should be controlled, smooth, and slow.
- Perform approximately 10 repetitions of the exercise.

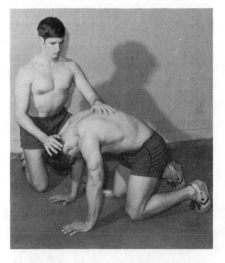

Neck extension: starting position.

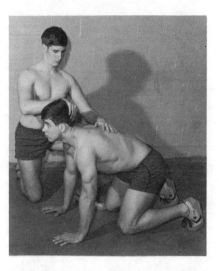

Neck extension: mid-range position.

NECK EXTENSION

Muscles used: Neck extensors

Starting position: Assume an all-fours position with your neck totally relaxed and your chin touching your chest.

Description of exercise: Lift your head upward and backward until your neck is fully extended and hold this position momentarily. Take approximately 4 seconds to complete each repetition.

Spotting: Your partner places his/her hand on the back of your head and gently applies pressure to stretch the neck muscles. As you raise your head, your partner should apply direct pressure to your head and vary the resistance throughout the exercise; recover to the starting position without any resistance being applied by your partner.

Points of significance:

- Take approximately 4 seconds to complete each repetition.
- Do not jerk your head. All movements should be controlled, smooth, and slow.
- Perform approximately 10 repetitions of the exercise.

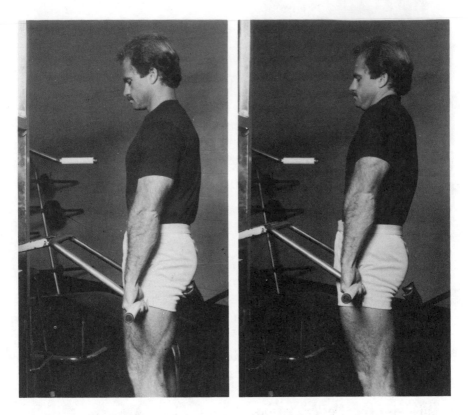

Shoulder shrug: starting position.   **Shoulder shrug: mid-range position.**

SHOULDER SHRUGS

Muscles used: Trapezius, shoulder

Starting position: Stand upright with your arms extended; hold the bar slightly wider than shoulder width with an overhand grip (palms facing you).

Description of exercise: Without bending your arms, raise your shoulder girdle a high as possible; pause momentarily and recover to the starting position.

13

NAUTILUS EXERCISES

by
Daniel P. Riley
Washington Redskins
and
John Donati

If you have access to Nautilus equipment, you can implement a selection of the following exercises into your program. The exercises involve all the major muscles of your body.* Whenever possible, you should perform the exercises in the following order:

1. Hip and back	11. Bent arm fly (Double Chest)
2. Leg extension	12. Decline press (Double Chest)
3. Leg press	13. Chinups (Multi-Exercise)
4. Leg curl	14. Dips (Multi-Exercise)
5. Hip abduction	15. Bicep curls (Curl-Tricep)
6. Hip adduction	16. Tricep curls (Curl-Tricep)
7. Lateral raise (Double Shoulder)	17. Neck flexion (4-way Neck)
8. Seated press (Double Shoulder)	18. Neck extension (4-way Neck)
9. Pullover	19. Shrugs (Neck and Shoulder)
10. Torso arm	20. Abdominal curls

*Most of the Nautilus machines currently available are included in this program. If you're interested in any machine which is not discussed in this chapter, we suggest that you contact the manufacturer.

LEG EXTENSION

Muscles used: Quadriceps.

Starting position: Sit on the leg extension machine with your feet hooked under the rollers; the back of your knees should be in contact with the front edge of the padded seat; lean back with your hands cupped (not making a fist) and grasp the hand grips; your head and shoulders should be back against the seat.

Description: Extend your legs forward and upward to a fully extended position; **pause momentarily**, then recover to the starting position. Do not let the weight plates being lifted return to the weight stack—this will allow your muscles to momentarily recover.

Points to emphasize:
- The same seat adjustment should be used each time the exercise is performed.
- You must reach the legs-extended position and pause momentarily for each rep. If you can't, the weight is too heavy or you have reached the point of failure.
- Do not lean forward while lowering the weight, stay back in the seat.
- Do not raise your buttocks off the seat while lowering the weight.
- If the Compound Leg machine is used, the leg press exercise should be performed immediately upon completion of the leg extension.

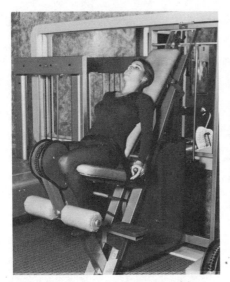 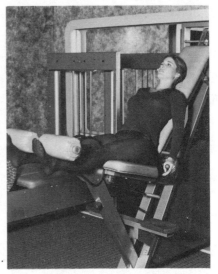

Leg extension: mid-range position.   **Leg extension: starting position.**

HIP AND BACK

Muscles used: Buttocks, lower back.

Starting position: Lie on your back on the Hip and Back machine with the ball and socket of your hip aligned with the axis of rotation of the Nautilus cam; your hands should grasp the stationary handles; your legs should be extended.

Description: Your right leg should remain stationary in the contracted position while your left leg moves backwards to the stretched position and then recovers to its starting position. Your left leg then remains in the contracted position while your right leg moves backwards to the stretched position and then recovers to its starting position.

Points to emphasize:

- Do not pull with your hands while raising the weight.
- The leg that remains extended should not move at all while the other leg is being exercised. If the leg remaining in the extended position moves at any time while raising or lowering the weight with the other leg, one or more of three factors are involved: the weight is too heavy, you are approaching failure, or you are coming back too far with the leg being exercised.
- Perform 8-12 reps with each leg.

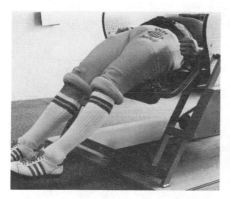 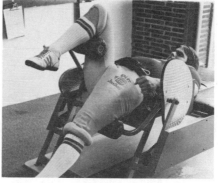

**Hip and back:
starting position.**

**Hip and back:
mid-range position.**

LEG PRESS

Muscles used: Buttocks, quadriceps.

Starting position: Sit with your feet on the leg press pedals; the center of your feet should be placed on the middle of the leg press pedals. The seat should be adjusted so that your legs are being exercised through a range of movement of 90° or less.

Description: Extend your legs until they are almost extended. Do not lock your legs—this will allow your muscles to recover momentarily. Next, recover to the starting position without allowing the weight plates being lifted to touch the weight stack which is not being lifted.

Spotting: Because this exercise is started in a position where there is a distinct mechanical disadvantage, the spotter can assist you to initiate the first repetition by pushing with his hands on the foot pedals of the leg press machine.

Points to emphasize:

- The seat should be in the same position every time the exercise is performed.
- If you get a headache while performing the exercise, you can relieve the headache by undertaking one or more of the following: don't squeeze your hands while grasping the hand grips (cup your hands); don't hold your breath; move the seat back until your headache disappears; perform the leg press first and the leg extension second; relax your face and neck; don't shrug the shoulders.
- Your buttocks should remain in contact with the seat throughout the exercise.

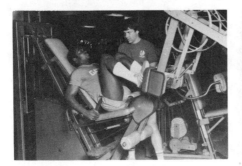

Leg press: starting position.

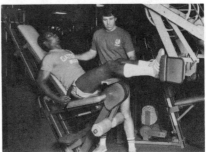

Leg press: mid-range position.

LEG CURL

Muscles used: Hamstrings.

Starting position: Lie face down on the Leg Curl machine with your heels hooked under the roller pads; your kneecaps should be positioned just off the edge of the pad, with your ankles flexed and your toes pointed toward your knees at all times.

Description: Flex your lower legs, pulling them upward and forward until they are at least perpendicular to the floor; pause momentarily, then recover to the starting position. Your ankles should remain flexed throughout the exercise.

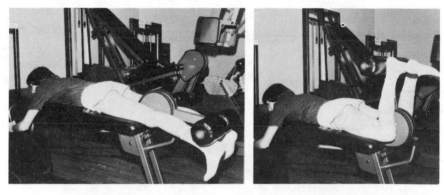

Leg curl: starting position.

Leg curl: mid-range position.

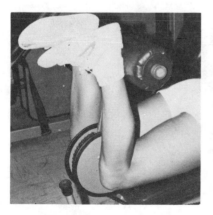

The proper position for your toes.

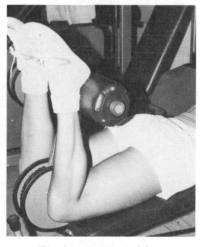

The improper position for your toes.

HIP ABDUCTION

Muscles used: Gluteus medius.

Starting position: Adjust the level on the right side of the machine until both movement arms are together; move the thigh pads to the outer position. Sit in the machine and place your knees and ankles on the movement arms. Your outer thighs and knees should be firmly against the resistance pads. Keep your head and shoulders relaxed against the seat back.

Description: Spread your knees and thighs to the widest possible position and pause; return slowly to the starting position and repeat.

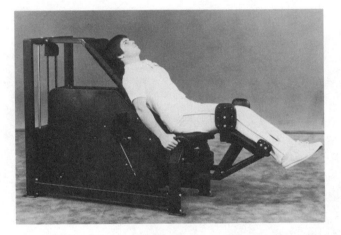

Hip abduction: starting position.

Hip abduction: mid-range position.

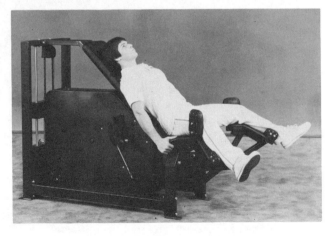

HIP ADDUCTION

Muscles used: Adductor magnus.

Starting position: Adjust the lever on the right side of the machine until the movement arms are as wide as comfortably possible. Move the thigh pads to the inside position. Sit in the machine and place your knees and ankles on the movement arms. Your inner thighs and knees should be firmly against the resistance pads. Keep your head and shoulders relaxed against the seat back.

Description: Press your knees and thighs smoothly together and pause; return slowly to the starting position and repeat.

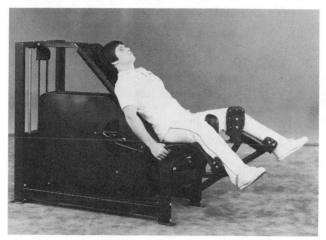

Hip adduction: starting position.

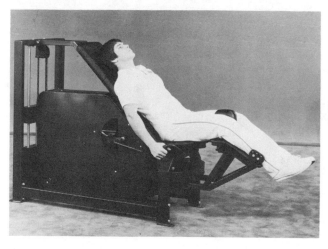

Hip adduction: mid-range position.

SIDE LATERAL RAISE

Muscles used: Deltoids.

Starting position: Sit with the ball and socket of your shoulders aligned with the axis of rotation of the Nautilus cam. Grasp the hand grips and place the back of your wrists against the pads; pull back on the hand grips. Your back should rest against the seat.

Description: Leading with your elbows until your upper arms make contact with the handles used for the seated press exercise, raise your arms upward; pause momentarily, then recover to the starting position.

Spotting: Once you complete the side lateral raise exercise, the spotter should change the amount of weight so that you can immediately initiate the seated press exercise.

Points to emphasize:

- Lead with your elbows and not with the hands; do not drop your elbows and push only with the hands.
- If your elbows are **pulled back** and your forearms are kept **parallel** to the floor, your deltoid muscles will be fully contracted when the elbows are just above parallel to the floor. The seat is adjusted correctly, if in this position the back of your arms just barely touch the seated press handles.
- Your legs should be kept on the seat with your feet crossed.
- Use the same seat setting each time the side lateral raise and the seated press exercise are performed. The same seat setting should be used for both exercises.

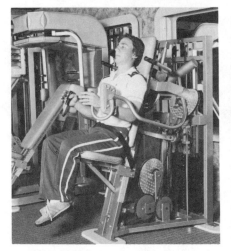

Side lateral raise: starting position.

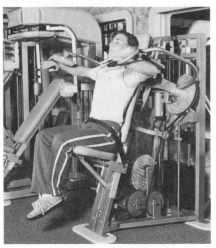

Side lateral raise: mid-range position.

SEATED PRESS

Muscles used: Deltoids, triceps.

Starting position: Sit with your hands grasping the seated press handles; rest your back against the seat pad.

Description: Extend your arms fully upward; pause momentarily, then recover to the starting position.

Points to emphasize:

- Upon completing the side lateral raise exercise, you should immediately initiate the seated press exercise.
- Do not arch your back.
- Do not remain in the locked out (mid-range) position.

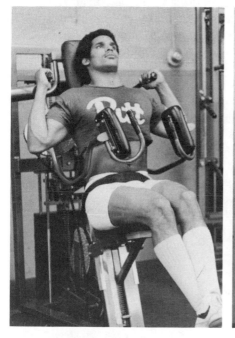 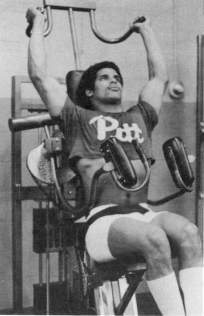

Seated press:
starting position.

Seated press:
mid-range position.

PULLOVER

Muscles used: Lats.

Starting position: Sit with the pullover bar resting against your waist; your elbows should be placed against the elbow pads; the sides of your hands should rest against the pullover bar (in a karate chop manner); your torso should be perpendicular to the floor; and the seat belt secured.

Description: Lower the weight allowing the pullover bar to move upward and backward to a stretched position; pause momentarily, then recover to the starting position.

Points to emphasize:

- Do not lean forward while raising or lowering the weight.
- Do not grab the bar; use the sides of your hands to hold the bar.
- Pause momentarily with the bar resting against your stomach each rep. If you cannot pause in that position, you either are using too much weight, threw the weight, or are approaching failure.
- Adjust the seat so that the ball and socket of your shoulders in the stretched position is aligned with the axis of rotation of the Nautilus cam.

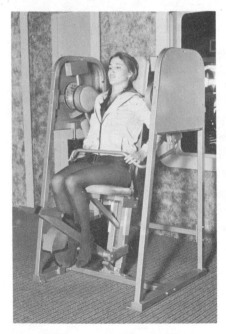 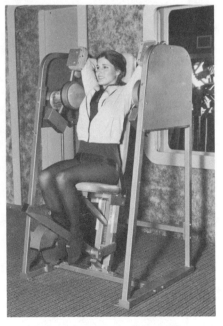

Pullover: starting position.   **Pullover: mid-range position.**

188

TORSO ARM

Muscles used: Lats, biceps.

Starting position: Sit with your arms extended; grasp the torso arm handles using an underhand grip. Your lats should be in the stretched position. The weight plates being lifted should not be touching the weight plates which are not being lifted. The seat should be lowered from the seat setting used for the pullover exercise.

Description: Pull the bar downward, drawing your elbows back; pause momentarily, then recover to the starting position.

Points to emphasize:

- Do not flex your wrists while pulling the weight downward. This act will force your forearm flexors to perform additional work and cause your forearms, not your lats, to reach the point of failure.
- Do not oversqueeze the torso arm bar. Oversqueezing will also cause the forearms to fatigue.

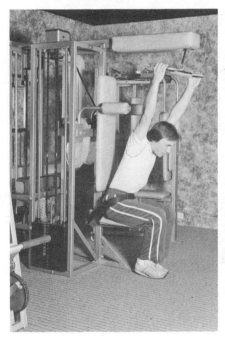 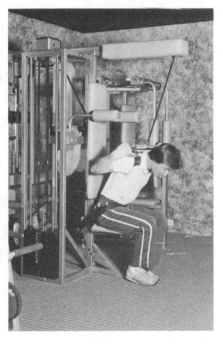

Torso arm:
starting position.

Torso arm:
mid-range position.

BENT ARM FLY

Muscles used: Pectorals.

Starting position: Sit on the Double Chest machine with your forearms resting behind and against the arm pads on the machine. Your thumbs should be hooked under the top hand grips (the hand grips should meet the junction of your thumb and index finger). Your elbows should be slightly higher than the ball and socket of the shoulders.

Description: Leading with your elbows, move your forearms forward until your pectorals are fully contracted; pause momentarily, then recover to the starting position.

Points to emphasize:

- Do not allow your elbows to leave the forearm pads; lead with your elbows throughout the exercise.
- Do not lean forward while raising or lowering the weight.
- Use the same seat setting every time the exercise is performed.

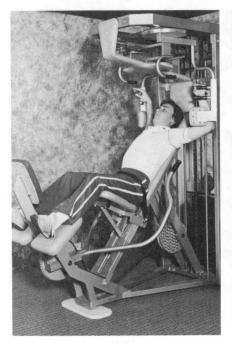

**Bent arm fly:
starting position.**

**Bent arm fly:
mid-range position.**

DECLINE PRESS

Muscles used: Pectorals, deltoids, triceps.

Starting position: Using the same seat setting that was used for the bent arm fly exercise, sit on the Double Chest machine with the decline press handles in the arms-extended position.

Description: Lower the weight, fully stretching the pectorals; pause momentarily, then recover to the starting position.

Spotting: The spotter should change the weight as soon as you complete the bent arm fly exercise so that you can immediately perform the decline press.

Points to emphasize:
- Do not rest in the locked out position.

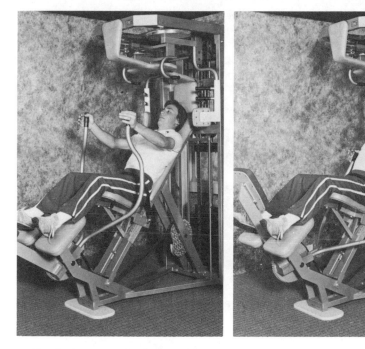

Decline press: starting position.   **Decline press: mid-range position.**

NEGATIVE-ONLY CHINUPS

Muscles used: Lats, biceps.

Starting position: Hang from the chin bar in a flexed-arm hanging position; use a just closer than shoulder width underhand grip; your legs should be bent to prevent your feet from touching the floor; your elbows should be pulled back.

Description: Walk up the stairs and assume a position with your chin over the bar; pause momentarily, then lower the body taking four seconds.

Points to emphasize:

- Keep your elbows pulled back.
- You should concentrate on gripping the bar only as tightly as is needed. Overgripping will cause your forearms to fail sooner than they should.
- When you assume the flexed-arm-hang position by stepping off the step, you should hold that position momentarily before lowering yourself.
- Adjust the height of the chin bar so that when you step off the steps, your chin will be over the bar; you should not have to jump to get over the chinning bar.
- A weight belt can be used to provide additional resistance.

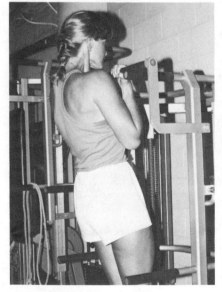 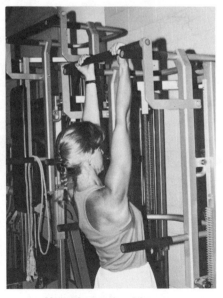

**Negative-only chinups:
starting position.**

**Negative-only chinups:
mid-range position.**

DIPS

Muscles used: Chest, shoulders, triceps.

Starting position: Assume an arms-extended position on the dip bars.

Description: Lower your body to a point where your upper arms are at least perpendicular to the ground; pause momentarily, then recover to the starting position. If you are performing negative-only dips, you should use the steps to recover to the starting position.

Points to emphasize:

- Make sure that you assume a fully stretched position at the mid-point of each rep.
- Do not rest in the locked out position.
- As you approach the point of muscular failure, be cautious that you do not allow your arms to collapse while in the arms-extended position.
- A weight belt can be used to provide additional resistance.

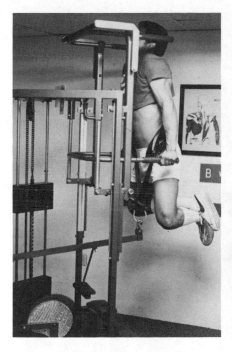

Dips: starting position.

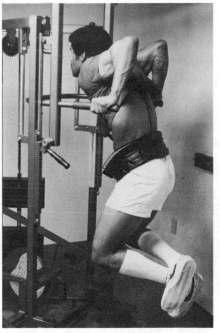

Dips: mid-range position.

BICEP CURLS

Muscles used: Biceps.

Starting position: Sit with a pad between your chest and the curl pad (this will keep your torso back in the machine and provide your biceps with a full range exercise). Your arms should be extended and your head and torso kept well back. Align your elbows with the axis of rotation of the Nautilus cams.

Description: Flex your arms, raising the weight to a position where your biceps are fully contracted; **pause** momentarily, then recover to the starting position.

Points to emphasize:
- Do not touch your chin on the bar in the contracted position. This will allow your biceps to rest momentarily.
- Do not let your elbows slide back and forth. They must remain stationary.

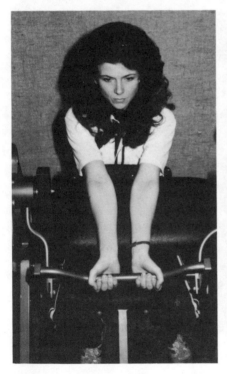

**Bicep curls:
starting position.**

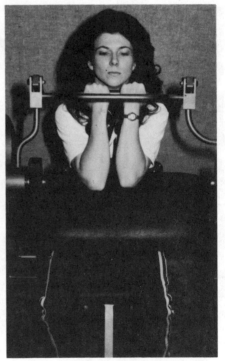

**Bicep curls:
mid-range position.**

TRICEP EXTENSION

Muscles used: Triceps.

Starting position: Sit with the side of your hands resting on the triceps extension pads in the stretched position. One or two pads may be needed to raise you to a position where your arms are parallel to the floor in the extended position. If you are too low in the seat, your arms will not be parallel to the floor in the extended position. A wooden bar can be placed between your hands to prevent them from sliding off the pads.

Description: Extend your arms completely; pause in the contracted position, then recover to the starting position.

Spotting: The spotter can assist you getting into and out of the machine by pulling the triceps extension bar over.

Points to emphasize:

- Use the side of your hands throughout the exercise. Do not roll your hands over and place your palms on the pads. Keep your hands in a karate chop position.
- Do not push with your fingers and wrists in the extended position. Force your **triceps, not** your wrist flexors, to completely extend the weight.

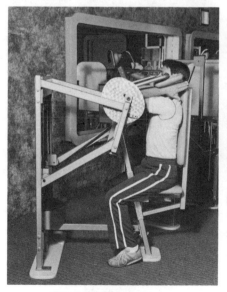

**Tricep extension:
mid-range position.**

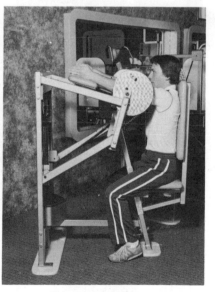

**Tricep extension:
starting position.**

NECK FLEXION

Muscles used: Neck flexors.

Starting position: Sit with your face against the two face pads, looking downward; grasp the two forward hand grips.

Description: Lower the weight so that your neck flexors are fully stretched; pause momentarily, then recover to the starting position.

Points to emphasize:

- All movements should be slow and controlled.
- Keep your torso erect and stationary. Do not allow your upper body to move backwards while lowering the weight. Your arms can be crossed to eliminate excess movement during the exercise by your torso.
- The same seat setting should be used every time the exercise is performed.
- If the correct seat setting is used, your face will not move or slide on the face pads.
- Two-and-one-half-pound plates should be used as additional increments. When you can perform 10-12 properly executed reps, you should add 2-1/2 pounds. For most individuals, a five-or-ten-pound increase may be too much.

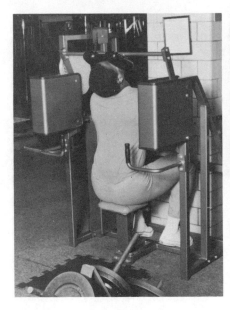

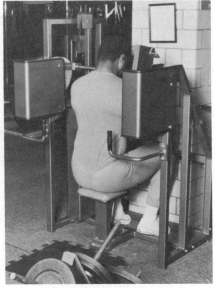

Neck flexion:
starting position.

Neck flexion:
mid-range position.

NECK EXTENSION

Muscles used: Neck extensors.

Starting position: Sit with the back of your head resting against the center of the two face pads; your torso should be erect and your head should look downward.

Description: Extend your head backwards, looking skyward; pause momentarily, then recover to the starting position.

Points to emphasize:

- Do not lean forward while the weight is being lowered (sit erect throughout the exercise).
- Tuck your chin toward your chest in the starting position to provide maximum stretching.
- The seat setting for the neck extension exercise will be lower than the seat setting used for the neck flexion exercise. The seat must be low enough so that in the contracted position, the bottom of the pads do not touch your trapezius muscles and prevent full range of movement.

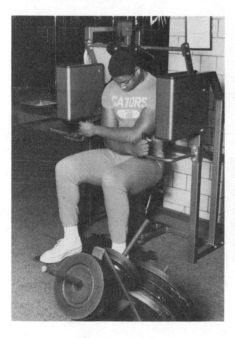 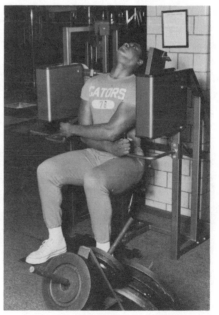

| Neck extension: | Neck extension: |
| starting position. | mid-range position. |

SHRUGS

Muscles used: Trapezius.

Starting position: Sit on the shrug machine with your forearms placed between the upper and lower pads; your palms should be facing skyward; your arms should be pushed forward so that your biceps are in contact with the upper pads (throughout the exercise); the back of your hands should be pushing downward against the lower pads to prevent your arms from being pulled back; your torso should be erect.

Description: Elevate your shoulder girdle as high as possible; pause momentarily, then recover to the starting position.

Points to emphasize:

- Do not lean backwards while raising the weight.
- Do not pull your arms backward; keep your biceps against the front side of the pads.
- You may need one or two additional pads (depending upon the length of your torso) to ensure stretching the trapezius muscles in the starting position. The weight plates being lifted should never touch the weight stack which is not being lifted until the exercise is completed.

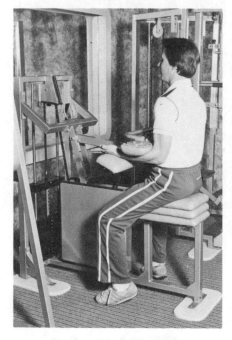 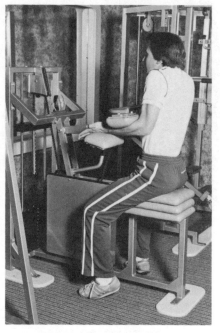

Shrugs: starting position. **Shrugs: mid-range position.**

ABDOMINAL CURLS

Muscles used: Rectus abdominis.

Starting position: Adjust the seat so the lower part of your sternum is even with the lower edge of the top pad; place your ankles behind the roller pads; spread your legs and sit erect; grasp the handles and keep your elbows high. Your shoulders and head should remain against the pad.

Description: Shorten the distance between your rib cage and your navel by contracting your abdominals; do not pull with your arms or lift up with your legs; pause in the contracted position; return to the starting position and repeat.

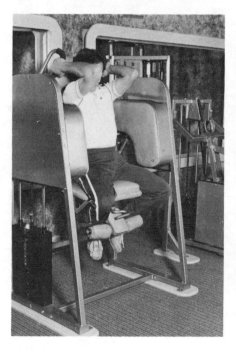

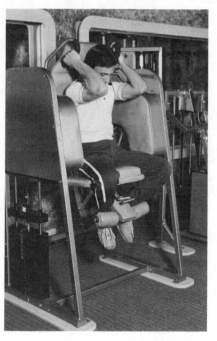

Abdominal curls:
starting position.

Abdominal curls:
mid-range position.

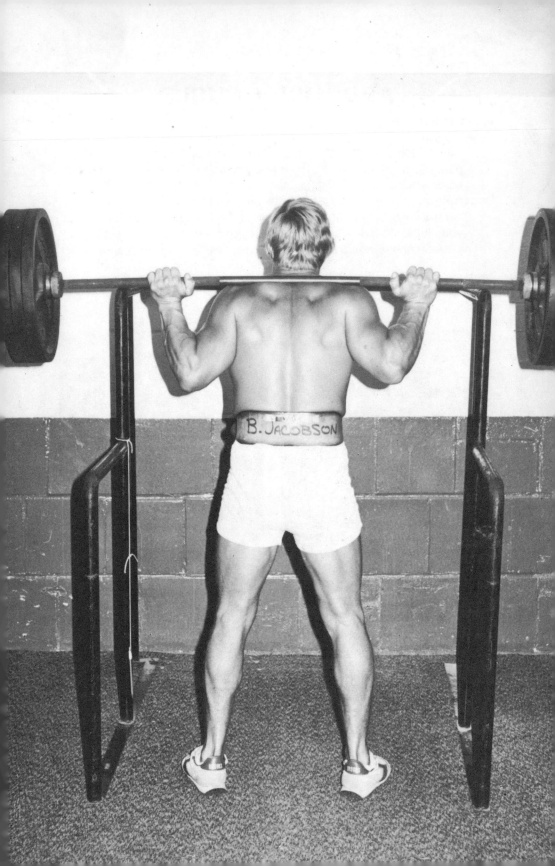

14

SYSTEMS OF TRAINING

by
Bert Jacobson
Head Strength Coach
Oklahoma Outlaws (USFL)

SPLIT ROUTINE

This is a workout that will consume a relatively short time from four to six times per week. The time in the weight room during each session is cut in half, but the frequency of times to work out is increased. The split routine divides the workout into two parts and allows the trainee to work out on four to six consecutive days. The most popular method of dividing the workout is to work your upper body Monday, Wednesday, and Friday and to work your lower body on Tuesday, Thursday and Saturday. If only five days are used, alternate so that your lower body is worked three times every other week. This is a very good means to develop strength. Be sure not to work the same body parts on two consecutive days.

ALTERNATE DAY ROUTINE

This type of system includes a total body workout every other day. Both the upper body and the lower body will be worked approximately two to three times per week. The duration spent in the weight room is increased but the number of times to work out per week is decreased. Usually a Monday, Wednesay, and Friday schedule is followed.

Whether a split or an alternate day routine is used, there are certain types of procedures that can be adopted to implement the routine. These are chosen according to the individuals involved and equipment available. Sections A-G offer an overview of several of the more popular procedures.

A.   Manual Resistance

This is the type of program many schools have gone to almost exclusively. It allows you to experience total muscle fatigue for every exercise encountered. The great advantage of this type of training is that each exercise is completed within 50 to 70 seconds. The training consists of both positive and negative fatigue for each exercise and can be done with either free weights or machines. With a reduced time factor involved, you can receive a total workout (legs, neck, and upper body) in less than forty-five minutes.

To begin the workout, you are paired with a partner. You and your partner apply the additional resistance to each other.

A weight is used that you can lift between six to eight repetitions before reaching positive failure. As positive failure occurs, your partner aids you in raising the weight as the exercise continues until you cannot resist in the negative phase of the lift.

It is important to note that during the primary repetitions of the lift, your partner applies resistance to the weight in the negative phase. The weight should be lowered by you to a count of four and raised to a count of three. The entire exercise should not exceed twelve repetitions. Again, positive failure should occur between six and twelve repetitions.

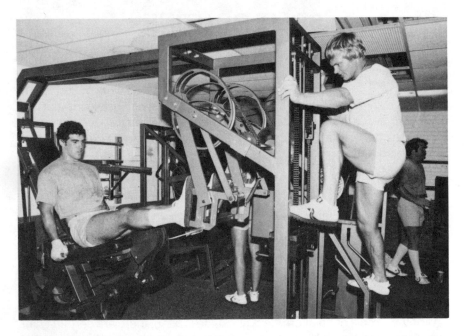

During the primary repetitions of an exercise in which manual resistance is being used, the partner applies resistance to the weight in the negative (lowering) phase.

For example, manual resistance while performing the bench press exercise would involve the following: you assume your position on the bench as your partner stands at the head of the bench. You begin by taking the barbell off the rack and holding it at full extension above your chest. Your partner puts his/her hands on the bar also, and begins forcing the bar down to your chest. You should resist the pressure by slowly letting the bar down to your chest to a count of four. When the bar touches your chest, your partner disengages from the bar and lets you push the bar out to full extension again. After six to eight repetitions, you should not be able to raise the weight by yourself. The exercise continues as your partner aids in the lifting of the weight. As the weight is returned to full extension, your partner again gives pressure to the weight while you resist. Note that toward the end of the exercise, less and less pressure needs to be applied by your partner. You should remember that a total effort should be given to every repetition. Manual resistance is certainly the most intense method of weight training available. You will achieve great results quickly. Exercises that involve pulling motions such as upright rows or curls are performed the same way. Your partner simply increases the weight by manual resistance.

During the pull up or dip exercises, when failure occurs, you merely use a bench to step up to the starting position, step off the bench, and resist your own weight against gravity. In the first few repetitions, your partner will manually pull you down. Manual resistance is not used for squats and stiff leg dead lifts.

Be sure that weights are recorded and increased as positive failure reaches eight repetitions. The weight you lift must be carefully documented so that you will use the proper weight the next time you work out.

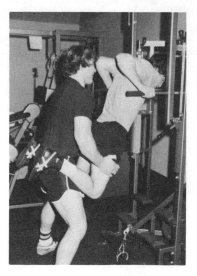

Manual resistance provides the most intense form of weight training available.

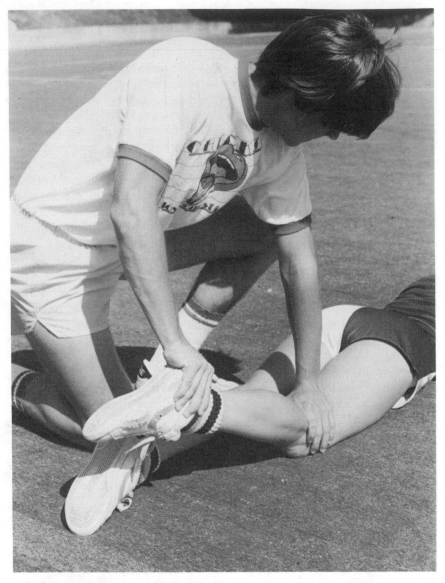

One of the advantages of manual resistance training is that substantial results can be quickly achieved.

(Editor's note: A complete description of manual resistance exercises for every major muscle group in the body can be found in the book, Maximum Muscular Fitness: Strength Training Without Equipment; written by Daniel P. Riley and published by Leisure Press: West Point, N.Y.; 1982.)

B. Circuit Training

A circuit involves a multiple station system. You begin at a particular station, complete one set of exercises, and move to another station, and then another, until the circuit is complete. Usually a measure of performance is to decrease the time it takes for you to complete the circuit doing a specific amount of weight for a determined amount of repetitions in a single set. A circuit looks like this:

Bench Press	10
Lat Pull	10
Military Press	10
Pull Ups	6
Sit Ups	10
Leg Press	10

C. Pyramid System

The pyramid routine is one that is favored by many body builders. It begins by working a specific muscle group using a relatively light weight so that about twelve repetitions can be performed. After each set, the weight is increased and the repetitions are decreased until only one or two repetitions can be performed. The weight is then progressively decreased after each set until twelve repetitions can again be performed.

EXAMPLE: Curls 12, 10, 8, 6, 4, 6, 8, 10, 12
    Bench 10, 8, 6, 4, 6, 8, 10

D. Superset

A set of exercises for one specific area is performed and immediately a set of exercises for the antagonistic muscles is performed. The number of sets can vary from three to six for each muscle group. The repetitions are usually limited to between eight and ten. An example of supersets is:

Bicep Curls	8
Tricep Extensions	8
Bicep Curls	8
Tricep Extensions	8

E. Tonnage System

This routine employs heavy weight for short repetitions. It will consist of between six and eight sets per muscle group. It is an excellent means of strength development but a poor means of developing muscle endurance. It is also a time consuming method.

EXAMPLE: Bench Press - 6 reps. 280 lb., 6 reps. 280 lb.,
    4 reps. 290 lb., 4 reps. 290 lb.
    2 reps. 300 lb., 2 reps. 300 lb.
    1 rep. 305 lb.

Repetition	1	2	2-3	3-4	4-5	5-6	6-7	7-8	8-10	12+
Percentage	95%	93%	90%	85%	83%	80%	78%	75%	70%	65%
Amount Lifted	285	280	270	255	250	240	235	225	210	195

*Based on 300 lb. Max.

An example of a percentage system based on a 300 pound maximum level of strength for this particular lift.

F.   Percentage System

This type of workout consists of using a specific amount of weight for each repetition. The weight to be used is determined by a percentage of your maximum strength for each lift. The number of repetitions performed will determine the weight to be used. The amount lifted should be based on your maximum recorded capability.

G.   Negatives

The lowering of the weight is considered the negative work of the exercise. The negative aspect of strength is the most powerful and the last to be fatigued. Many believe that the key to strength development is negative work. Negative exercises should be done by slowly lowering the weight. The weight should be more than the maximum amount that you can lift in the positive phase. Some individuals believe that at least 150% of the maximum should be used. Of course, you need a training partner on each exercise to help you raise the weight back to the starting position in the negative phase.

15

MOTIVATING ATHLETES*

by
Chet Fuhrman
Strength and Conditioning Coach
United States Naval Academy

Before you can motivate anyone, you must first be highly motivated your-self. There is no systematic approach to motivation. Each person must develop his/her own individual approach that best suits his/her personality and the situational conditions. Having the ability to motivate others is a great asset and, as a close friend once told me, it is something that no one can take away from you.

Athletes, and people in general, are usually motivated to do things that they feel are important to them. Lifting weights is not enjoyable for many athletes. I feel certain that every coach in the country has a number of athletes who dislike or even dread the idea of being in the weight room. Therefore, coaches must make their athletes aware of the importance of proper strength training. From the head coach to every assistant coach, the athlete must receive feedback that strength training is important and a vital part of the total athletic program. Through positive feedback and rein-forcement, all staff members can get involved in the strength training pro-gram. Your athletes must be sold on the importance of strength training. By taking this particular approach, your athletes may see new reasons for their participation.

---

*Editor's note: This chapter examines methods that coaches can use to motivate their athletes in the weight room. Although it is directed at coaches, readers who are not coaches will undoubtedly be able to apply some of the points to their own particular needs and interests. At the time this chapter was written, Mr. Fuhrman was employed as the Strength and Conditioning Coach at Weber State College.

TECHNIQUES FOR MOTIVATING YOUR ATHLETES

● The best way I have found to motivate athletes to work in the weight room is first to explain to them **why** it is important for them to be there. If you were to tell your athletes that the only reason for them to lift weights is to get bigger and stronger, some of them might not feel that it is all that important. However, if you tell them that higher levels of muscular fitness will make them less susceptible to injuries—especially in key areas such as the neck, knee and shoulder—they may become more motivated.

Another reason that athletes should engage in a strength training program is that it will improve their level of performance. Certainly, there is not a bonafide athlete on any team anywhere that does not want to excel. Higher levels of performance may be the basis for greater levels of personal commitment by the athlete towards strength training.

● Try to make your strength training facility as pleasant as possible. It helps to have the room nicely painted, carpet on the floor, mirrors on the walls, and music the athletes enjoy listening to. After reading this, you may have two concerns: 1) that this type of atmosphere sounds a little too luxurious for a weight room; and 2) where and how you might obtain all these materials.

The first problem is less serious once you realize the magnitude of the positive feelings that are generated by a positive atmosphere. Nice paint, carpet, mirrors and music may seem to be luxuries, but are in actuality major contributors to the positive atmosphere of a weight room. As a result, these amenities can also serve as chief contributors to the process of motivation.

If you are concerned about where and how to obtain all of these things, you should remember that there are many different ways to get something if you really need it. For example, it might be a good project for an art class to paint the room and perhaps put murals of different types of athletes on the walls. Someone in town might be willing to donate an old (or even new) carpet to the facility. Maybe some of the athletes have mirrors they could donate, or perhaps they could organize some fund raising activity to purchase them. Another suggestion would be to make contact with your school's audio-visual department and request that they lend your facility some type of radio or cassette player.

Another way to make the atmosphere more positive and to get some involvement from another department would be to have a photography class from your school take pictures of your athletes lifting. Then, display the pictures on the walls of the weight room (people like to see themselves in a picture). You might even consider giving the athletes the photos of themselves at the end of the year.

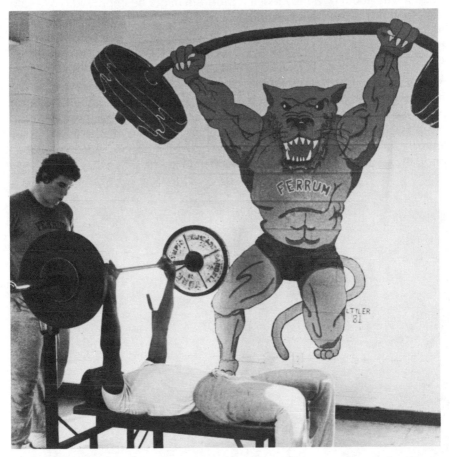

One of the best ways to motivate athletes is to let them motivate each other by peer awareness.

- Incorporate variety in your program. Make your program fun. If your program becomes monotonous, your athletes may become bored and eventually completely turned off. You should periodically review and evaluate your program. This review should include some feedback from the athletes themselves about how they feel the program might be improved. To break the monotony of the workouts, perhaps you could bring your team together at the end of every couple of sessions for a ten to fifteen minute session of basketball, volleyball, fun relays or some other activity. You will probably find that your athletes will leave that day with a more positive attitude.

- Use verbal encouragement at all times. Much of the progress of an athlete depends on how often someone pays attention to that athlete, and how often he/she receives information concerning his/her performance progress. Try to be as positive and reinforcing as you can at all times. I believe in the saying, "Make me feel good and I will produce." Accentuate the good things as often or more, if possible, than the negative things.

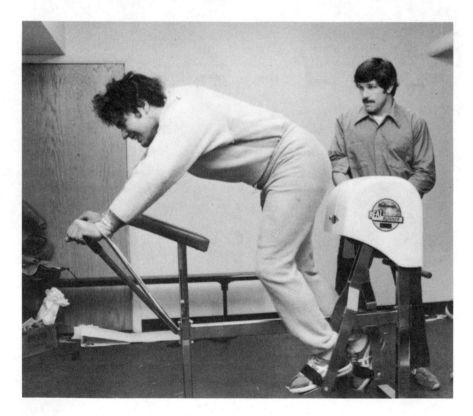

Use verbal encouragement at all times.

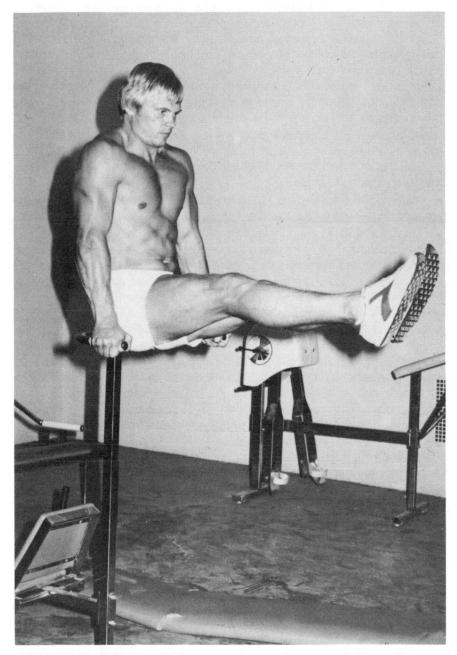

Incorporating variety into your program is an excellent motivational technique.

- Use attendance as a tool for motivation. As a coach, you know that having your athletes in attendance is half the battle. Even if on a particular day an athlete is not giving one hundred percent to a task, the effort of attendance is at least better than nothing. Possible ways to increase an athlete's desire to attend a workout session are readily available. Large visual attendance charts are usually good motivators. Coloring in the days that the athletes have worked out is frequently a good indication of how strong the athlete is, how strong the class is (i.e., sophomore, junior, senior etc.), and how strong the entire team will be. Attendance can also be the basis for individual awards. Such awards are particularly valuable since they can be obtained by any member of the team regardless of his/her size or team status, etc. Attendance awards give athletes a readily attainable goal which they can be motivated to achieve.

- Tap other sources, such as fellow coaches, teachers, parents and the athletes themselves, to help motivate your athletes. When others get involved, your athletes are not only hearing from you. They receive the benefits of considering different perspectives—perspectives which at the least might make them more confident, more secure, or at least more aware. If other coaches and influential people encourage the athletes to participate in the strength training program, it would also help make the job of the strength coach (coordinator) a lot easier.

Enlighten the parents of your athletes that a good strength training program is important to their children and explain why. Organize a "parent's night" and show the parents some of the things their sons and daughters are doing. I have found that most parents are concerned with the safety of their children and thus, since strength training reduces the chances of someone being injured, would support a program of strength training. Once parents are educated about the true value of strength training, they can prove to be a strong motivational force on the athlete.

Probably the best way (other than the first one I mentioned) that I have discovered to motivate athletes is to let them motivate each other by peer awareness. The seniors on the team, the team captains, or those whom the team respects as leaders can be fruitful sources of peer motivation.

- Remember that motivation involves constant effort. You might ask, "When is the best time to motivate my athletes?" I have found great success motivating athletes before, during, and after a workout. By using many of the aforementioned motivation tools and personalizing these tools to suit your situational variables, you may be able to psych up your athletes for the workouts, reinforce them throughout, and thus make the experience more positive for everyone involved. It is generally a good idea, during or at the end of a workout, to give your athletes some constructive criticism. This is the time that they are most aware of what they are doing. Accordingly, your comments may be particularly helpful at this time.

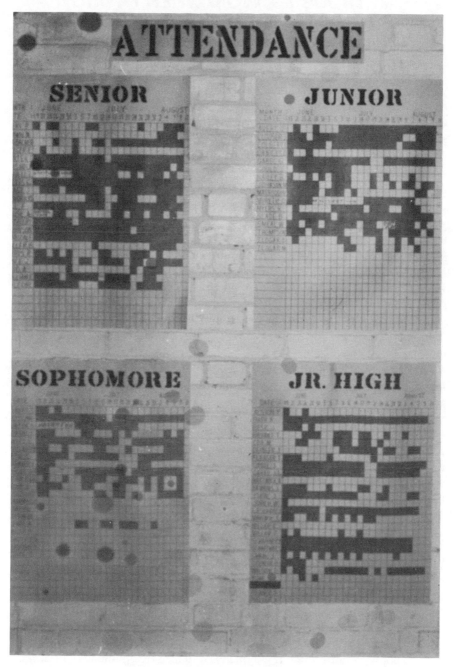

Use attendance as a motivational tool.

METHODS TO AVOID WHEN TRYING TO MOTIVATE YOUR ATHLETES

● Do not threaten or embarrass your athletes. If you threaten or embarrass them by any means, you risk the possibility of losing them from your program. Be patient with them. Take your time in winning them over. It may take weeks or even months to accomplish this, but the rewards of having loyal and dedicated athletes is well worth any efforts you might make.

● Do not try to motivate your team **only** as a group. Group motivation is important, but is secondary to motivating athletes on a one-to-one basis. By responding solely to the needs of the group, you might ignore the individual needs of many or all of your athletes. Remember that not all athletes can be motivated by the same techniques. Each athlete responds to different kinds of motivational cues. This is where you, as the coach, must be flexible in your motivational skills.

● Do not compare your athletes to one another. A coach may tell his team, "O.K. team, Leo has worked harder than anyone on the team this summer. He has increased his bench press by one hundred pounds. So everyone work as hard as Leo and you'll look as big and be as strong as he is." Leo, however, may be genetically gifted—an individual who is very muscular and very well-developed. Most of your team members will know that no matter what they do, they will never look like Leo. Only compare your athlete to one person: him or herself.

● Do not have "pound clubs" for your team. Many high schools and colleges use this as a big motivational tool. For example, the three hundred pound bench club, the six hundred pound squat club, etc. In these clubs, your goal as a coach is to have all or as many of your players as possible in each pound club. If you were to actually evaluate how many of your athletes were in each of the pound clubs, you would probably find that only a small percentage of your team would appear on the list.

For every athlete you might turn on using this system, you would probably turn another one off. The majority of your athletes know that their name will never appear on the chart and won't even bother with it. Those who might be so motivated by the desire to achieve a certain level of performance that they might compromise the proper execution of doing the exercise, such as bouncing, jerking or throwing the weight. Since such people probably need very little motivation anyway, it would seem that in the final analysis, the practice of "pound clubs" is not a very productive motivational tool overall.

● Do not attempt to use motivational trickery. If you tell your athletes one thing and then do another, you may lose their trust and respect. You will probably find much better success motivating your athletes by using a rational approach rather than a gimmick approach. Being totally honest with your athletes will better enable you to gain their confidence and respect.

- When there is a time you feel it necessary to discipline an athlete, express your concerns to the athlete in private. If other team members become unnecessarily involved, it may cause a strain on your relationships with the athletes and thus have a negative effect on the positive motivational atmosphere you have worked hard to build. Also the team member(s) might feel very embarrassed in front of their peers.

- Do not give trophys or awards to those who lift the most. If you do, you will find that only a small percentage of your team will be rewarded (as in the "pound clubs"). Remember that the quarterback in your program (if it is football, for example), can only bench press one hundred pounds. Even though he is a great athlete, he will never receive an award because he will never be the strongest member of the team. Give incentive awards that everyone can obtain.

SUMMARY

Motivation is a year round process and should be practiced on a daily basis. It is imperative for you, as a coach, to demonstrate to your athletes that you have an interest in them, and that you care for their welfare. This attitude should not exist only in the weight room. Rather, it should penetrate the walls of the weight room and exist in every aspect of coach-athlete interaction. Motivational contact outside the strength training facility is equally, if not more, important than that which occurs inside the facility. If you have the athletes highly motivated **before** they enter the weight room, your job will be made easier as a result once they are actually in the weight room.

Remember, be positive in everything you do. Enthusiasm is contagious!

Motivation is a year round process and should be practiced on a daily basis.

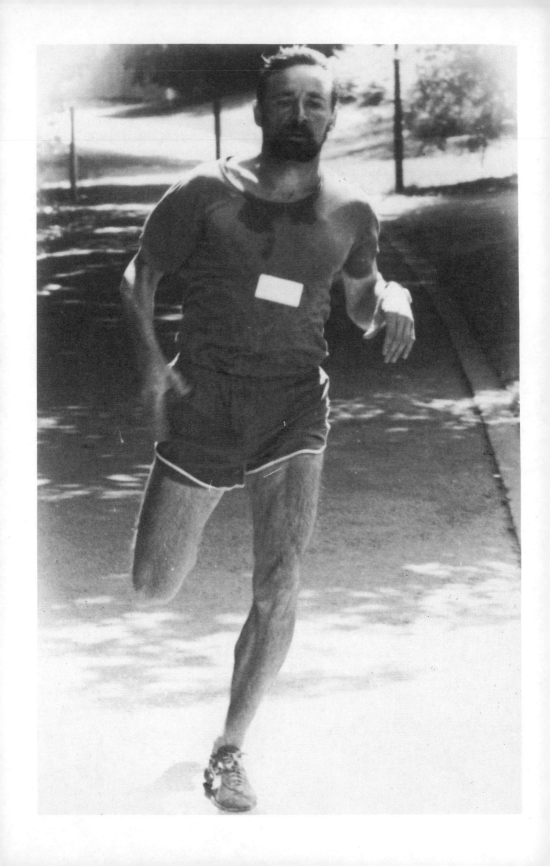

16

AFTER WORKING THE REST IS EASY*

by
E. C. Frederick and
J. E. Welch

(Editor's Note:)

*This article first appeared in *Runner's World Magazine* (December 1975) and is reprinted by permission of the publisher. Although the article deals with the importance of adequate amounts of rest for individuals involved with running, the principles are also extremely important for individuals who train with weights. Without an appropriate rest between training sessions, the individual achieves a less-than-optimal level of improvement.

Unfortunately many coaches and athletes continue to progress with the quantity of exercise being performed totally disregarding the body's ability to recover from exercise. The accepted practice by most coaches is to increase the amount of exercise (to be performed by the athlete) as the level of fitness improves. However, the body's ability to recover from exercise is totally ignored.

The body is only capable of recovering from a specific amount of exercise. To exceed this expenditure of energy will not allow the body to fully recover from the exercise. If this overexpenditure of energy continues, the level of fitness of the athlete will gradually decrease. At this point the coach would rationalize by saying that the athlete has reached a "plateau" or a period of "staleness." The standard procedure would then be to prescribe a brief rest period.

The coach and athlete must realize that exercise is performed to stimulate an increase in fitness.

If an athlete overloads the muscles properly and allows adequate time to recover, he should stimulate an increase in fitness (regardless of how small) each and every workout. If an increase is not recorded, the athlete is performing too much exercise, not allowing adequate time to recover, or not properly overloading the muscles involved.

In the area of strength training it has been supported that the quantity of exercise can be drastically reduced while producing better results. It should be the goal of the coach and athlete to stimulate the greatest increase in fitness with the least amount of exercise. A new philosophy may be, "It is not *how much* exercise but *how* you perform the exercise that counts."

A coach involved in any activity in which the athlete is trying to improve the level of fitness should evaluate the revolutionary concepts of quality vs. quantity exercise now being utilized in the area of strength training. It is my contention that most athletes could decrease the quantity of exercise considerably and continue to produce the same results. The implication might be that most athletes perform too much exercise not allowing the body to fully recover. By performing less exercise the athlete might recover more readily from the exercise.

His doctors were upset at his determination to race. It appeared pointless. Not even Emil Zatopek could hope to overcome the debilitating effects of his hospitalization in time to compete.

Zatopek had been bedridden for some two weeks with a serious stomach ailment. It seemed impossible that he could be competitive after missing two weeks of training and in such a weakened state. Nevertheless, his determination won out and within an hour of his discharge he was aboard a plane for Brussels and the 1950 European Championships. The rest is history.

Zatopek nearly lapped second place Alain Mimoun in the 10,000 meters and captured the 5000 by a 23-second margin. Distance running historian Peter Lovesey has termed his victories "the most decisive double long distance victory in any major international championship." It seems only logical to add that Zatopek's effort was all the more amazing when we remember the two weeks of training that he missed. Or is it?

Most modern coaches and runners would have us believe that everyday training is essential for maximal performances. Equally well touted is the dogma that points to continuous hard work as the only path to high level running achievement.

We have serious doubts about the supposed truth underlying these ideas. If this training dogma was based on fact, then how could Zatopek, for example, achieve his decisive victories following two weeks of bedrest? A "fluke" would be the answer of the hard trainers. Or perhaps it could be explained away by Zatopek's overwhelming superiority or by speculating poor preparation on the part of his competitors.

These criticisms might be reasonable if the Zatopek story were an exceptional one. The startling thing is that the pattern is not unique. Similar incidents have happened time and again.

Two years ago, Dave Bedford surprised the track world by running a world record for 10,000 meters. The surprise was not that Bedford had run that fast but he had done it with only minimal training. Bedford had been nursing a hamstring injury which hampered his running. Instead of his characteristic high mileage weeks, which sometimes pushed 200 miles, he had been barely averaging 25 miles for a three-month period.

Bedford did have the benefit of three weeks of accelerated training following this light period. But few serious proponents of the hard-training dogma would consider three weeks enough to put the athlete at a world record peak. The answer has to be in his **rest**.

Dick Taylor, Commonwealth Games 10,000-meter winner, was in a similar situation. Torn ankle ligaments allowed him only three weeks of hard training before the Games.

Another Commonwealth Games competitor, 800-meter silver medalist, Mike Boit, also had little training before the New Zealand competition. After

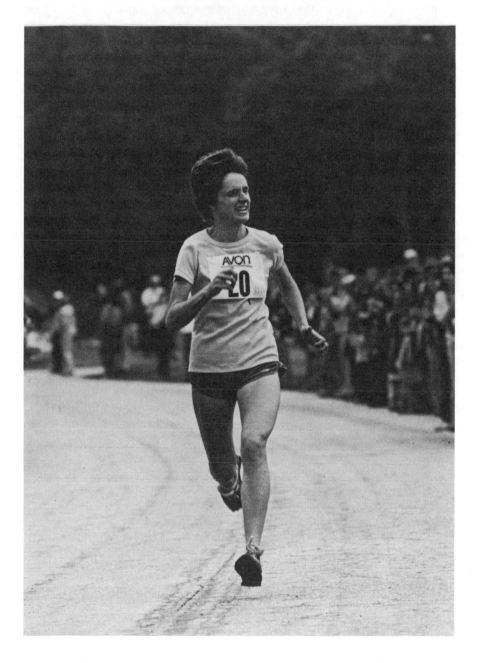

"Most modern coaches and runners would have us believe that everyday training is essential for maximal performances."

a month's layoff, he trained only two weeks before running 1:44.4 in the final.

Another not so dramatic example is supplied by Craig Virgin. Virgin was unable to train for more than a month due to severe tendonitis. In early February he began training again, and on February 11 he ran an outdoor double. While his times of 4:12.5 and 8:51.0 are not world class, they were, at that time, strong performances for Virgin.

Emil Puttermans missed 14 days of training six weeks before the Munich 10,000 final yet he ran 27:39 to win the silver medal.

Dave Wottle missed 31 days of training between the Trials and the Munich Olympic Games, averaging only about four miles a day during that period. Yet he had the strength to come from behind in the 800-meter final and win the most exciting race of the Games.

The examples go on and on at all levels of competition. The pattern repeats itself again and again...Hard work and rest = success.

We can learn from these examples. They teach us that our ideas of what constitutes an effective training program need some revision. We need to take a closer look at the function of rest in a running program. But, before doing that, we need some perspectives on the use of rest in modern training programs.

Overtrained runners are much more common than undertrained runners. Observing this aspect of the problem, you would think that runners were generally uninformed about the importance of rest. Ironically, this does not seem to be the case.

Engage a group of runners in a conversation about rest, and you'll find that most of them agree that rest is important. Most will also agree that they probably don't get enough of it. Perhaps a number of them will even admit to having given it some serious thought. But in all likelihood, only a very few will have ever done anything about it.

Rest is a lot like stretching exercises in that respect. A lot of lip service is paid to its importance, even to its necessity. But few runners actually incorporate it into their training programs. We are creatures of habit, and our bad habits (or lack of good ones) are firmly entrenched.

Realizing the worth of something, intellectually, does not guarantee that a constructive change will result. Cognition is one phenomenon, application another. Most often, the bad situation will persist and the new realization will fade into the background.

This seems particularly true when dealing with ideas that relate to the body and health. How many people do you know who wish they could lose a few pounds or give up smoking but "just can't"?

The reason so many runners have neither stretching nor rest built into their training programs can only be apathy and/or negligence. The thing that keeps them from caring is largely an attitude we have developed about natural things and their relationship to the will.

What enforces this attitude is a lack of any clear conception of why rest is needed and what rest does. Further, many runners have no idea of how much rest is needed or just how to go about it.

Our Western concept of the path to success doesn't include rest. Instead, the formula contains liberal doses of persistent hard work aimed at overcoming resistance—the resistance supplied by natural physical limits, intellectual capability, financial constraints, etc. It seems like it is always man against nature...man overcoming himself. When we get a headache from overstressing, do we stop and rest? No, we take a pill and forge on. The body is just another obstacle on the path to success. All too often, we see it as the object of conquest rather than cooperation.

This brings to mind an interesting story about the first ascent of Mount Everest. There are some enlightening parallels with competitive running.

When Edmund Hilary and Tensing Norgay returned from their successful climb, they had different ideas about what had taken place. New Zealander Hilary spoke triumphantly of conquering the mountain. Norgay, a Sherpa, saw things differently. He stated humbly, "The mountain and I together attained the heights."

More often than not, runners see their bodies as Hilary saw Everest—as another obstacle in their paths. When a runner does well, the impression one gets is that success has come in spite of the body, rather than because of it.

It appears that many (if not most) runners have lost touch with the simplest of realities. They have lost sight of the fact that it is the whole organism which achieves and not just the power of will. Most runners are too busy conquering themselves with high-mileage weeks to see the profound significance of this idea.

If we could only realize that we can gain more (in the largest sense) by cooperating with the body than by trying to conquer it, everything would fall into place. We would begin to see running as a means to develop the body to make maximum performance possible. Words like "nurture, coax, and develop" would replace "thrash, push, and force." The necessity of rest would become dramatically obvious.

Running is an exercise in destruction. Each time we run, we tear ourselves down. Muscle tissue is torn. Mitochondria, the powerhouses of the cells, swell grotesquely. Metabolic wastes accumulate. Blood-sugar levels drop. Dehydration occurs and, along with it, excessive losses of electrolytes upset the delicate balance required for efficient muscle and nerve function. We become overheated. Muscle glycogen is depleted. And as the intensity and/or duration of the workout increases, this damage becomes more pronounced.

In the period between runs, the body attempts to recover and to rebuild.

Torn muscle is repaired, new mitochondria are formed, metabolic wastes are flushed out of the system, and blood-sugar levels are restored. We rehydrate and replace lost electrolytes. Any damage to muscles and to the nervous system due to hyperthermia (high body temperature) is repaired. Glycogen is replenished.

These two phases—destruction and regeneration—together constitute conditioning. And the two can never be separated if a conditioning program is to proceed in a positive direction.

In any program of running, then, the body is systematically broken down and rebuilt. And each rebuilding leaves the body a little stronger than before. These incremental increases amount to the development of a progressively stronger body capable of more and faster running. That is, if it is done right.

If the body is not allowed to complete the rebuilding phase of training for lack of time (rest) or materials (nutrition), then the destruction will eventually exceed the body's ability to repair itself. Conditioning will proceed at a slower rate or not at all. In extreme cases, conditioning can actually deteriorate.

On the other hand, if the breakdown phase (the stress) is not optimal, then progress is also retarded. Since we have all become experts at the "stress" phase of training, nothing needs to be said about effective training methods. But the rebuilding phase—let's call it "regeneration"—does need some elucidation.

Some aspects of the regenerative phase take longer than others. All depend, to a certain degree, on the intensity and duration of the stress. For example, glycogen depletion, mitochondrial destruction and extensive muscle tissue damage all take about 48 hours to be completely reversed. Eating properly, getting plenty of rest and a little exercise seem to promote regeneration. Still the time period needed to completely return to the status quo is well over 40 hours.

To understand how this information fits into a running program, we need to juggle different intensities and durations of runs with the frequency of runs.

First of all, no one runs all day every day, so we have, say, 21 to 23 hours of non-exercise time during each day to recover from the physiological havoc created by a daily run. It should be obvious that the greater amount of time spent in intensive rest (e.g., sleep), the more effective the rest time is. It should be equally obvious that the more and faster we run, the more there is added to the regenerative load.

This regenerative load is the product of the speed and distance of workouts, and is also influenced by the quality and quantity of rest during the same time period. We can, therefore, regulate this load by controlling the relationship between our daily dose of destruction and our daily capacity to regenerate.

Let's say we take a hard 20-mile run in the afternoon of day one. If we do nothing on days two and three but rest and recuperate, we should be completely regenerated by the afternoon of day three. But few runners would be willing to do no running for such a period of time. So they are going to contribute to the regenerative load by running during this recovery time. If, however, they do only light workouts, get more rest than usual, and eat a diet rich in carbohydrates, protein and vitamins and minerals, they should regenerate on schedule. Or possibly they will need 72 hours to recover rather than the usual 48-hour period.

By tuning into such subtle body signs as stiffness and soreness, lack of energy, cravings for sweets, etc., it is possible for a runner to determine the period required for rebuilding from a particular workout. Workouts, rest and diet can then be adjusted to promote quick and total regeneration.

However, if runners do the opposite, continue hard workouts and make no concessions in the life-style, they will be delaying recovery from the hard run. Indeed, if high-intensity training is maintained continually, then the body never catches up with the regenerative load and eventually staleness and overstress symptoms will result.

In this way, workouts can be varied in intensity and duration from day to day to promote regeneration. Running hard or long only every 48 hours seems to be optimal. In between workouts should be short and/or easy, and one's life should be adjusted to maximize regeneration. Plenty of sleep is certainly important, but what one does with the waking hours is equally so.

This "cycling" of workouts is nothing new. Enlightened students of distance running, like Bill Bowerman and Tom Osler, have been preaching it for years. Its efficiency at producing optimal training effects has been proven time and again by the high proportion of world-class runners who have flourished on this type of program. So there should be little doubt that this type of training schedule is effective.

Much has been written about the structure and application of hard-easy training programs, so in all likelihood we wouldn't be able to contribute anything worthwhile. An area that does need to be developed, however, is the application of rest in this type of program. It is just as important as the running phase, and just as capable of being refined and perfected to produce maximal effects. Let's take a look at some regenerative techniques with an aim to maximizing our gains from this phase of conditioning.

Rest can be divided into two types: "passive rest" and "active rest." Passive rest is what we normally do, or actually don't do. In short, passive rest is inactivity. We do nothing in particular to promote rest, but instead give nature time to run its course. Passive rest certainly is important and effective. It has its place in a program of regeneration.

But there are other things we can do which will enhance regeneration and will multiply the effectiveness of rest. We would lump these activities under the heading of active rest. In other words, we are doing things to more effectively utilize the regenerative effects of rest.

After a hard run, things like light stretching, meditation, a sauna or a massage will cause regeneration to proceed more quickly than it would if we simply took a nap. These sorts of activities are regeneration promoting. Liberal doses of these activities can quicken and deepen healing, and thereby enhance the rebuilding of the body after a destructive run.

Yoga-type stretching exercises have been shown to stimulate circulation in all areas of the body but particularly in the exercised areas. There is also an enhancement of oxygenation of the tissues, not to mention the physical effects of the stretches on the muscle fibers themselves.

Meditation has been studied by a variety of researchers, and the majority of them have found it to be an intense form of relaxation and rest. The physiological state achieved in meditation is thought to be deeper even than sleep.

Sauna baths and steam baths are cleansing and often produce an intense relaxation, a relief of tension. Swimming and massage have similar relaxing qualities and have the added effect of promoting deep circulation.

These activities also have a soothing effect on the psyche, something which we have neglected so far, but something which is of equal or greater importance than the physical factors we've mentioned. We can regenerate a psyche which has been damaged or overworked by a long or hard run using the same positive approach we've taken in healing the body.

Do something unusual. Take a walk somewhere you've never been before, read something different, sit in a bus station and watch the world in action, catch a Walt Disney movie, take a long drive over a back road, walk in the rain, visit the ocean, go to a museum, make love (not necessarily in that order, nor one after another). In short, do something that will increase your awareness, stimulate you, generate new interests and ideas. It is just as important to have a fresh, healthy interest in your running as it is to have a sound body to do it with.

Bedford, Zatopek, et al., have stumbled upon the secret of this relationship. They have all followed long months of intense work with extended rest and then gone on to achieve superlative performances.

Their long months of steady intense work with only minimal regeneration produced a maximal stress load accumulated over time. The result was either sickness or breakdown beginning a period of enforced rest. During this prolonged rest period, their bodies were given the time and materials to completely rebuild—to adapt to the maximal stress which they had accumulated during months of intense training. In short, the body had time to catch up. The results were impressive.

Actually, what they were doing was no more than an extended version of what every runner should be doing constantly. Using the running-regeneration cycle on a day to day basis is a much more efficient way to accomplish the same goal—maximal adaptation.

Even the most conscientiously designed balance of running and regeneration is bound to produce an accumulation of stress over a long period of time. For this reason, runners should cultivate non-running rest periods from time to time.

For example, Emil Puttemans at least once a year has a period in which he does no running at all, he overeats, gets a little sloppy, becoming the antithesis of his normal self. Puttemans claims that these "rest" days are the most important part of his annual training pattern.

Ron Hill used to take at least a week's "vacation" during which he ran two daily workouts—two miles in the mornings and two in the afternoons.

Although the idea of not running for even a day can generate tremendous anxiety in certain runners, we don't believe their fears are well founded. After all, look what it did for Zatopek and Bedford.

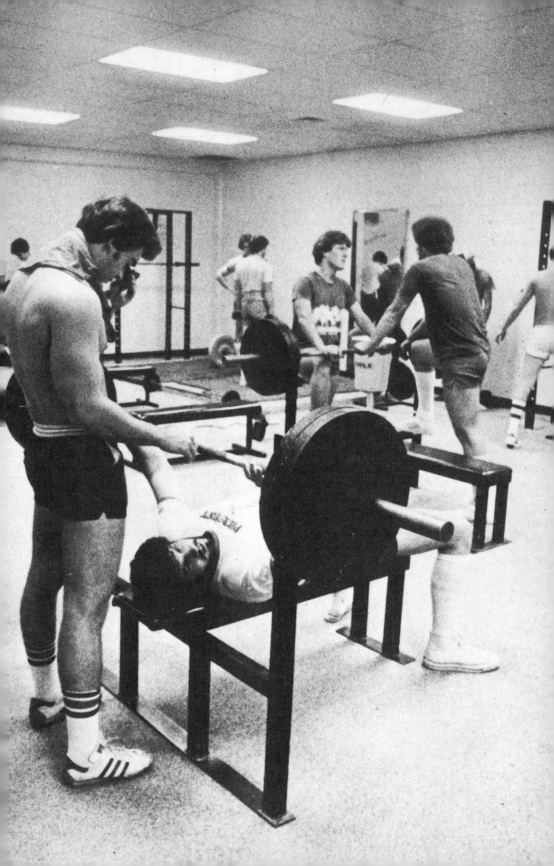

APPENDIX A

TEACHING STRENGTH TRAINING

by
Daniel P. Riley
Washington Redskins

This chapter is designed to provide an instructor with the basic information and guidelines needed to teach a strength development-weight training class at either the high school or the college level. The objective of this chapter is to provide an instructor with a reference and guideline to facilitate the preparation and organization of a course in strength development. It is of course obvious that the facilities, class size, duration of the class, and level of interest, will affect the structure of the course. Keep in mind, however, that even the most basic course must include a minimum amount of technical information. Without this pertinent data the course will be ineffective and objectives cannot be accomplished.

There is a growing interest in the area of strength training both on the high school and college level by athletes and non-athletes alike, including men and women. The time has arrived for physical education to provide students with the professional instruction required in this area.

The era of the student-athlete visiting the local gym to obtain information on how to best increase muscle strength and mass must end. This responsibility should be assumed by the physical educator.

The information that is obtained from the local gym or health club is often inaccurate and hand-me-down in nature. Seldom is this information based on scientifically sound training principles. It is usually information based upon the philosophy of the resident weightlifter or bodybuilder.

Although students can increase their strength by utilizing information disseminated in the local gym, this information is usually not the most efficient or scientifically accurate information available. Unfortunately, the young enthusiast relies upon this inaccurate information and eventually develops very poor training habits and incorrect techniques which in turn carry over and are very difficult, indeed almost impossible, to break.

To the benefit of everyone involved with sport and athletics, the body of knowledge relating to muscular development has finally caught up with and surpassed the information (which was primarily empirical in nature) previously known only by the bodybuilder and the weightlifter.

One of the main focal points of the physical education curriculum has always been to provide students and athletes with the most accurate information available on how to get and stay in shape. Unfortunately, very few physical educators possess either practical experience or a high level of interest in the area of strength training. Because of a general lack of interest by educators in strength training, students are denied the professional instruction they should receive. In general, such instruction is generally unavailable elsewhere.

There is a strong demand for information on how to properly organize, initiate, and sustain a strength development program. Physical educators should therefore prepare themselves to meet this demand. Since student interest in strength training frequently originates when the individual is in high school, physical educators at this level should give particular attention to this responsibility.

THE IMPROPER APPROACH

Unfortunately, the primary objective of most strength development classes is to "attempt" to increase the strength of the student during the course of instruction. More class time is usually spent trying to keep students busy or active while doing very little to prepare them with the ability to independently function on their own when the class is completed. During most strength training classes, the teaching of pertinent information and proper training techniques is frequently sacrificed for class participation. Circuits are arranged to provide the instructor with the ability to "herd" students into a class and periodically blow a whistle while students rotate around a series of exercise stations. While such a method may keep students busy (and in the end may be the only method to facilitate mass participation), it usually accomplishes very little in the way of stimulating an increase in either knowledge or strength.

Some of the disadvantages of the circuit approach are:
- It does not deal with the needs of the individual.
  a. Very often barbells with fixed weights are used.
  b. This may provide too much weight for one student and not enough for another.
- Upon termination of the class, you may not have this specific circuit to train on.
- An instructor will not always be present to blow a whistle (you must learn to function independently).
  a. The circuit approach may not prepare you with the ability to organize a program on your own.

Some of the limitations that exist with trying to stimulate strength gains during the course of instruction are:

- Irregular class schedules.
  a. The frequency of training may be too irregular to effectively stimulate significant strength gains.
- The duration of the course from beginning to end may not provide adequate training time to obtain marked improvement.
- Inadequate facilities in conjunction with overcrowded classes provide very poor training conditions.

Many instructors structure their course in such a way that students anticipate significant gains in muscle strength and mass upon completion of the teaching unit. These attitudes are fostered when pre-measurements are taken for muscle girth, bodyweight, maximum weight and repetitions on specific exercises and performance on selected tests (vertical jump, pushups, etc.). The students (and sometimes the instructor) become disillusioned, disappointed, and discouraged when significant gains are not obtained on post-measurements at the end of the course.

Instructors and students should realize that in most situations, a student will not significantly increase muscle mass and strength in an overcrowded class using inadequate facilities, which meets twice-a-week.

Many students also approach a strength training class with the "crash-course-philosophy" in mind. These individuals believe that such a course will develop them to their maximum potential and that they will never have to train again upon termination of the class. It should be emphasized that in most instances, muscular development is a long range proposition. It takes a considerble amount of time (with ideal training conditions) to make significant gains. Training should continue after the course has ended to obtain significant gains in muscle mass and strength. Due to the many limitations of most strength development classes, an instructor should encourage his/her students to train after the course is terminated if they wish to make significant gains in muscular fitness.

THE PROPER APPROACH

In a properly structured strength development class, one of the primary considerations should be to provide each student with enough information so that he/she is capable of organizing a sound, functional, and efficient program.

Instructors must strive to obtain the proper balance between lecture and practical work (involving the actual lifting of the weights during class time). The compromise between lecture and practical work will obviously vary with the class size, number of lessons, and the facilities available. Keep in mind that there is a minimum amount of time that must be spent on the theoretical, factual aspects of strength training. Students must be exposed to the necessary technical information to thoroughly understand the most basic elements involved in program organization.

The end product must be a student who is capable of independently interacting with all aspects of program planning and execution. Such students will be capable of independent interaction if they possess specific practical and cognitive skills.

Practical skills that should be obtained during the course of instruction should include the following:

- Properly perform at least one exercise for each of the major muscle groups in the body utilizing both conventional free weight equipment (barbells and dumbbells) and the Universal gym. These two are the types of equipment the student will probably have the greatest access to upon completion of the course.
- During the practical work, each student should obtain a starting weight for each of the exercises discussed in class and record both it and the repetitions performed on the workout data card. This provides the student with the information needed to begin training on a regular basis.
- Every student should become familiar with the proper execution and lifting techniques of each exercise to include the following:
  a. Properly raising the weight without using momentum or jerky movements.
  b. Learn to emphasize the lowering of the weights.
  c. Become familiar with and experience high intensity exercise.
  d. Proper spotting, breathing, grips, stance, etc.

Upon completion of the course, your students must be independently capable of organizing, initiating, and continuing a strength training program that will increase their strength and muscle mass to their maximum potential, utilizing the conventional equipment they may have available. To accomplish this, your students should be capable of the following cognitive skills:

- Organize a strength development program that is based on scientific principles and not on hand me down information.
- Identify the major muscle groups in the body.
- Know what the function of these muscles are during exercise. This knowledge provides students with the ability to observe a movement or activity and identify the primary muscles being used.
- Properly manipulate the strength training variables so that maximum strength gains can be obtained.

If you have modified the behavior of your students so that they are capable of the practical and cognitive skills previously discussed, you can be assured that they will leave your class with the knowledge and ability to continue a functional and progressive program on their own.

LESSON PLANS

This section presents a course outline with lesson plans to accommodate a 20 lesson unit in strength development-weight training. The structure and content of this outline can be monitored or altered to meet the demands of your particular teaching situation.

The format of each lesson plan is structured in the following manner:

   I.   **Question and review**
   II. **Lecture material**
   III. **Demonstration and critique**
   IV. **Practical work**

During "**I. Questions and review**", the instructor entertains questions from the students on the reading assignment, previous lessons, or pertinent information relevant to the course.

During "**II. Lecture material**", the instructor discusses the information outlined in the lesson plan for that class (additional information can be supplemented by the instructor if he so desires). It is my opinion that every student needs all of the information outlined in the lesson plans to follow.

During "**III. Demonstration and critique**", the instructor can request a student to perform the prescribed exercise for that class with the student emphasizing the following:

- major muscles used to perform the exercise
- prime mover
- starting position
- description of the exercise
- spotting
- breathing
- grip
- additional information that might facilitate the performance and safety of an exercise

This can be a graded exercise which would be a percentage of a student's final grade. Preparation, performance, and accurate information should be your basis for grading your students. This will also force your students to prepare before they come to class which can save you valuable class time and insure class participation and preparation. Upon completion of the student demonstrator's presentation, you and the class can critique the performance and provide additional information if needed.

During "**IV. Practical work**", all students should attempt to properly perform the exercise previously demonstrated by a student and critiques by you. This method allows each student to perform an exercise immediately after having been given instruction on the proper training techniques. This block of time also provides you with the opportunity to observe your students while they perform the exercises. You should pay strict attention to the execution and technique of your students' performance.

Student teams can be organized to perform these exercises. The number of students in each team will depend upon the amount of equipment available. In a high school situation where the equipment may be inadequate, you must emphasize proper form. This can be accomplished by actually supervising a student through a set of each one of the exercises to be discussed in class.

When there is an adequate amount of equipment, each student should strive to obtain two primary objectives during the "**practical work**" portion of the class.

- Learn and develop the proper techniques to perform each of the exercises correctly.
- Determine the correct starting weight for each of the exercises discussed in class.
  a. A proper starting weight is a weight in which the student can only perform 8-12 properly executed repetitions.
  b. Most students will stop exercising before they have reached that point of momentary muscular failure. You should, therefore, encourage your students to continue the exercise or find a starting weight in which they will fail between 8 and 12 repetitions.
  c. You must emphasize to the students that it will probably take a few sets (and possibly a few classes) before they actually determine their proper starting weight on each exercise (initially the weight may be too heavy or too light).
  d. Eventually when more time becomes available (either during or after class), a student may use this information and not waste time deciding what the proper starting weight should be.
  e. Once the starting weight has been determined, each student should record the amount of weight and the number of repetitions he/she performed so that there will be no difficulty in trying to recall how much weight should be used once he/she has the opportunity to perform the exercise on a regular basis.

There are a variety of workout data cards that can be used. You can modify the card to best meet the needs of your particular situation. Your data card should have space to include the exercises performed, the weight and number of repetitions of each exercise, the date, and if desired the amount of time taken for each workout. A sample workout data card for recording necessary information is illustrated on the next page.

During most of the classes, a new exercise should be added. The student can simply add the name of each exercise on the card as the course progresses. The card should be large enough to accommodate all of the exercises you eventually expect the students to be able to perform.

Due to the nature of strength training as an activity, it is recommended that you try many different methods to make the practical work as enjoyable as possible. Additional motivation may be needed initially to generate a sincere interest in many of the novice or beginning students. Very often training facilities are located in basements that are dark, damp, and aesthetically unattractive. This type of environment could demotivate even the most avid enthusiast.

The environment you provide for your class could be the catalyst needed to stimulate an immediate interest in strength training. You can provide a more enjoyable and aesthetically pleasing atmosphere by having a clean, well lit facility. Music is also an added attraction which is thoroughly enjoyed by most students.

The teaching unit described in the following section has lesson plans for 20 lessons. If your teaching unit is more than 20 lessons, you can decrease the amount of lecture material in each lesson and increase the amount of time devoted to practical work.

NAME Riley, Dan			CLASS		SECTION 1A
DATE	5/17	5/19	5/21	5/24	5/26
EXERCISE					
*Leg Press	170 lbs. 9 reps	170 lbs. 11 reps	170 lbs. 10 reps	170 lbs. 12 reps	175 lbs. 8 reps
*Bench Press	150 lbs. 10 reps	150 lbs. 12 reps	155 lbs. 9 reps	155 lbs. 10 reps	—
*Biceps Curls	40 lbs. 10 reps	40 lbs. 11 reps	40 lbs. 11 reps	—	—
*					
Total workout time	17 min.	19 min.	18 min.	—	—

A sample workout data card.

LESSON 1

I. Question and review period
    A. N/A

II. Lecture material
    A. Administrative procedures:
- Class policies.
- Grading.
- Uniform.

    B. Course objectives:
- to provide the students with enough information so that they are capable of organizing a strength training program.
- learn and develop proper lifting techniques.

    C. Outline the standard operating procedures for each class:
- first there will be a question and review period of reading assignments and previous lessons.
- the instructor will then lecture on pertinent information from the daily reading assignment.
- upon completion of the lecture, a student will be selected to demonstrate an exercise and explain the proper methods and techniques of performing the exercise.
- the instructor and class will then critique the student's performance and explanation of the exercise.
- if facilities allow, the class will divide into many teams (the number of students in each team will depend upon the amount of equipment available).
  - a. the students then attempt to properly perform the exercise previously discussed by the instructor.
  - b. emphasis should be placed on proper techniques and trying to determine a correct starting weight.
- the three previous steps should be repeated until each of the exercises for that particular class have been discussed.
- all remaining class time should be spent performing exercises that have been discussed in previous classes.

    D. Discuss benefits of strength training:
- strength.
- muscle endurance.
- power-speed of movement.
- CR fitness.
- flexibility.

    E. Proper training techniques:
- full range exercise.
- positive work.
- negative work.

- reaching the point of momentary muscular failure between 8 and 12 reps.
- proper supervision to stimulate maximum gains (train with a buddy).

F. Muscles of the legs and buttocks (refer to muscle chart):
   - buttocks.
   - quadriceps.
   - hamstrings.
   - calves.

G. Discuss the location and the primary function during exercise of the above muscle groups.

III. PRACTICAL WORK
   A. None.

IV. READING ASSIGNMENT
   A. The effects of a strength training program.
   B. Muscles of the legs and buttocks (refer to muscle chart).
   C. Fundamentals and techniques-intensity.
   D. Grips.
   E. Exercises:
      - hip and back.
      - squat.
      - leg press.

LESSON 2

I. QUESTION AND REVIEW PERIOD
   A. Entertain questions on reading assignment, previous lesson, or pertinent information relevant to the course.

II. LECTURE MATERIAL
   A. Fundamentals and techniques:
      - safety.
      - spotting.
      - breathing.
      - sweat suits.
   B. Grips:
      - overhand.
      - underhand.
      - alternate.
      - false.
   C. Intensity.
   D. Review major muscles of the legs and their primary function during exercise.

III. DEMONSTRATION-CRITIQUE
   A. Student demonstration of the barbell squat exercise.

      B. Instructor critique and explanation of the exercise.

IV. PRACTICAL WORK
- A. Student teams will attempt the following:
  - properly perform the barbell squat exercise paying strict attention to execution and proper lifting techniques.
  - determine a proper starting weight and record the weight and repetitions on their data workout card.

V. A. Student demonstration of the leg press exercise (if equipment is available).
- B. Instructor critique and explanation of the exercise.

VI. PRACTICAL WORK
- A. Student teams will attempt the following:
  - properly perform the leg press exercise paying strict attention to execution of proper lifting techniques.
  - determine a proper starting weight and record the weight and repetitions on their data workout card.

VII. READING ASSIGNMENT
- A. Fundamentals and techniques:
  - record workout data.
  - exercise the antagonists.
- B. Exercises:
  - leg extension.
  - leg curl.
  - heel raise.

LESSON 3

I. QUESTION AND REVIEW PERIOD
- A. Entertain questions on the reading assignment, previous lessons or pertinent information relevant to the course.

II. LECTURE MATERIAL
- A. Fundamentals and techniques:
  - record workout data.
  - exercise the antagonist.
- B. Review the location and primary function of the quadriceps, hamstrings, and calves.

III. DEMONSTRATION-CRITIQUE
- A. Student demonstration of the leg extension exercise.
- B. Instructor critique and explanation of the leg extension exercise.
- C. Student demonstration of the leg curl exercise.
- D. Instructor critique and explanation of the leg curl exercise.
- E. Student demonstration of the heel raise exercise.
- F. Intructor critique and explanation of the heel raise exercise.

IV. PRACTICAL WORK

A. With the remaining class time, the student teams should attempt the following:
- perform the exercises discussed in this class and determine the starting weight for each and record it on data card.
- perform the exercises discussed in previous classes and record the weight and repetitions on the workout data card.

V. STUDY ASSIGNMENT
A. Advantages and disadvantages of the various methods of training:
- normal exercise.
- negative only exercise.
- negative accentuated exercise.
B. Pectorals:
- location and function during exercise.
C. Exercises:
- bench press.
- incline press.
- decline press.

LESSON 4

I. QUESTIONS AND REVIEW PERIOD
A. Entertain questions on the reading assignment, previous lessons, or pertinent information relative to the course.

II. LECTURE MATERIAL
A. Advantages and disadvantages of various training methods.
- normal exercise.
- negative only exercise.
- negative accentuated exercise.
B. Pectorals.
- location.
- function during exercise.

III. DEMONSTRATION-CRITIQUE
A. Student demonstration of the bench press exercise.
B. Instructor critique and explanation.
C. Student demonstration of the bench press exercise with dumbbells.
D. Instructor critique and explanation.

IV. PRACTICAL WORK
A. Student teams will attempt the following:
- properly perform the bench press exercise with a barbell and a dumbbell paying strict attention to execution and proper technique.
- determine a proper starting weight and record the exercise, amount of weight and number of repetitions on the data card.

V. DEMONSTRATION AND CRITIQUE
   A. Student demonstration of the incline press with a barbell and dumbbells.
   B. Instructor critique and explanation.
   C. Demonstration of the decline press with a barbell and dumbbells.
   D. Instructor critique and explanation of the exercise.
VI. PRACTICAL WORK
   A. Student teams should attempt the following:
      • perform the decline and incline press with a barbell and dumbbells and record the necessary data on the workout card.
      • use remaining class time to perform the exercises discussed in previous classes.
VII. STUDY ASSIGNMENT
   A. Equipment.
   B. Exercises:
      • bent-arm pullover.
      • bent-arm fly.

LESSON 5

   I. QUESTION AND ANSWER PERIOD
      A. Entertain questions on reading assignment, previous lessons, or information relevant to the course.
  II. LECTURE MATERIAL
      A. Equipment:
         • discuss the nomenclature, proper use, and function of the most common pieces of conventional free weight equipment.
 III. DEMONSTRATION AND CRITIQUE
      A. Student demonstration of the bent-arm pullover exercise with a barbell and dumbbells.
      B. Instructor critique and explanation of the exercise.
      C. Student demonstration of the bent-arm fly exercise.
      D. Instructor critique and explanation of the exercise.
 IV. PRACTICAL WORK
      A. Student teams will attempt the following:
         • perform the bent-arm pullover exercise with a barbell or dumbbells paying strict attention to execution and technique.
           a. determine a starting weight and record on the data card.
         • use remainder of class to perform the exercises discussed in previous classes.
         • record all weight and repetitions on data card.
  V. STUDY ASSIGNMENT
      A. Step I: How to organize a program:
         • program considerations.

- organize a program that is:
  a. sound.
  b. functional.
  c. efficient.
- prerequisites.

LESSON 6

I. QUESTION AND ANSWER PERIOD
  A. Entertain questions.
II. LECTURE MATERIAL
  A. Step I: How to organize a program:
  - program considerations.
  - organize a program that is:
    a. sound.
    b. functional.
    c. efficient.
  - prerequisites.
III. DEMONSTRATION AND CRITIQUE
  A. Review exercises that students may not be properly performing.
IV. PRACTICAL WORK
  A. Student teams should attempt the following:
  - use the remainder of the class to perform as many of the exercises previously discussed as possible.
  - record all data on the workout card.
V. STUDY ASSIGNMENT
  A. Step II: How to organize a strength development program:
  - repetitions.
  - sets.
  - workload.
  - time interval between exercises.
  B. Deltoids:
  - location.
  - primary function during exercise.
  C. Exercises:
  - seated press
  - upright row.
  - side lateral raise.

LESSON 7

I. QUESTION AND REVIEW
  A. Entertain questions.
II. LECTURE MATERIAL
  A. Step II: How to organize a strength development program.
  - repetitions.

- sets.
- workload.
- time interval between exercises.

  B. Deltoids:
  - location.
  - primary function during exercise.

III. DEMONSTRATION AND CRITIQUE

  A. Student demonstration of the seated press exercise with a barbell and dumbbells.

  B. Instructor critique and explanation of the exercise.

IV. PRACTICAL WORK

  A. Student teams should attempt the following:
  - properly perform the seated press exercise paying strict attention to execution and technique.
  - determine the proper starting weight and record it on the data card.

V. DEMONSTRATION AND CRITIQUE

  A. Student demonstration of the upright row.

  B. Instructor critique and explanation of the exercise.

  C. Student demonstration of the side lateral raise.

  D. Instructor critique and explanation of the exercise.

VI. PRACTICAL WORK

  A. Remaining class time can be spent performing the upright row, side lateral raise, and the exercises discussed in previous classes:
  - strict attention should be paid to execution and technique.
  - record all exercises, weight and repetitions of each exercise on the workout data card.

VII. STUDY ASSIGNMENT

  A. Step II (cont'd): How to organize a program:
  - frequency of workout.
  - adaptation energy.
  - order of exercise.
  - exercises to be performed.

  B. Trapezius:
  - location.
  - primary function during exercise.

  C. Exercises:
  - shoulder shrug.

LESSON 8

  I. QUESTION AND REVIEW PERIOD

  II. LECTURE MATERIAL

A. Step II: How to organize a strength development program:
- frequency of workout.
- adaptation energy.
- order of exercise.
- exercises to be performed.

B. Trapezius:
- location.
- primary function during exercise.

III. DEMONSTRATION AND CRITIQUE
A. Student demonstration of the shoulder shrug exercise.
B. Instructor critique and explanation.

IV. PRACTICAL WORK
A. Student teams should attempt the following:
- perform the shoulder shrug exercise paying strict attention to execution and proper technique.
  a. determine a proper starting weight and record on data workout card.
- remaining class time can be spent performing exercises discussed in previous classes.
  a. record all weights and repetitions of each exercise performed on the data workout card.

V. STUDY ASSIGNMENT
A. Review previous assignments.

LESSON 9

I. QUESTION AND REVIEW
II. LECTURE MATERIAL
A. None
III. DEMONSTRATION AND CRITIQUE
A. Preview specific exercises not being properly performed by the students.
IV. PRACTICAL WORK
A. Student teams will attempt the following:
- properly perform as many of the exercises discussed in previous classes as possible.
- strict attention should be paid to execution and technique.

V. STUDY ASSIGNMENT
A. Muscle physiology:
- muscle structure.
- muscle contraction.
- strength curve.
- muscle soreness.
- variable or accommodating resistance

LESSON 10

I. QUESTION AND REVIEW PERIOD

II. LECTURE MATERIAL

A. Muscle physiology:
- muscle structure.
- muscle contraction.
- strength curve.
- muscle soreness.
- variable resistance or accommodating resistance.

B. Lower back muscles:
- location.
- primary function during exercise.

III. DEMONSTRATION AND CRITIQUE

A. Student demonstration of the deadlift and stiff-legged deadlift exercise.

B. Instructor critique and explanation of the exercises.

IV. PRACTICAL WORK

A. Student teams will attempt the following:
- properly perform the stiff-legged deadlift exercise emphasizing execution, technique, and determining a starting weight.

V. DEMONSTRATION AND CRITIQUE

A. Student demonstration of the goodmorning exercise.

B. Instructor critique and explanation.

C. Student demonstration of the hyperextension exercise.

D. Instructor critique and explanation of the hyperextension exercise.

VI. PRACTICAL WORK

A. Student teams will attempt the following:
- properly perform the goodmorning and hyperextension exercise emphasizing execution and technique.
  a. record all weight and repetitions on the data card.
- use remaining class time to perform the exercises discussed in previous classes.
  a. record all weight and repetitions on the data card.

VII. STUDY ASSIGNMENT

A. Equipment:
- isokinetic machines
- Nautilus machine

B. Latissimus dorsi
- location.
- primary function during exercise.

C. Exercises:
- chinups.

- lat pulldowns.
- bent over rowing.

LESSON 11

 I. QUESTION AND REVIEW PERIOD
 II. LECTURE MATERIAL
   A. Equipment:
   - isokinetic machines
   - Nautilus machines
   B. Latissimus dorsi:
   - location.
   - primary function during exercise.
 III. DEMONSTRATION AND CRITIQUE
   A. Student demonstration of the chinup exercise.
   B. Instructor critique and explanation.
 IV. PRACTICAL WORK
   A. Student teams should attempt the following:
   - properly perform one set of chinups.
     a. normal or negative only.
     b. emphasis should be placed on execution and proper technique.
     c. record weight and repetitions on data card.
 V. DEMONSTRATION AND CRITIQUE
   A. Student demonstration of the bent-over rowing exercise with a barbell and dumbbell.
   B. Instructor critique and explanation.
   C. Student demonstrations of the lat pulldown exercise with the overhand and the underhand grip.
 VI. PRACTICAL WORK
   A. Student teams will attempt the following:
   - properly perform the bent over rowing exercise.
   - proper perform the lat pulldown exercise.
   B. Remaining class time can be spent performing exercises discussed in previous classes.
 VII. STUDY ASSIGNMENT
   A. Review.

LESSON 12

 I. QUESTION AND REVIEW PERIOD
 II. LECTURE MATERIAL
   A. None.
 III. PRACTICAL WORK
   A. Student teams should attempt the following:

- remaining class time can be spent performing as many exercises as possible that have been discussed in previous classes.
    a. emphasis should be placed on execution and proper techniques.
    b. record all exercises, weight and repetitions, on data card.

IV. STUDY ASSIGNMENT
   A. Genetic factors affecting strength development.
   B. Triceps:
      - location.
      - primary function during exercise.
   C. Exercises:
      - French curl.
      - triceps extension.
      - dips.
      - L-seat dips.

LESSON 13

   I. QUESTION AND REVIEW PERIOD
   II. LECTURE MATERIAL
   A. Genetic factors affecting strength development:
      - bodytypes.
         a. ectomorph.
         b. mesomorph.
         c. endomorph.
      - biomechanical advantages.
         a. length of lever.
         b. insertion point of the muscle.
      - physiological advantages
         a. neuromuscular efficiency.
         b. quality of fibers.
         c. quality of belly length.
   III. DEMONSTRATION AND CRITIQUE
   A. Student demonstration of the French curl exercise.
   B. Instructor critique and explanation.
   IV. PRACTICAL WORK
   A. Student teams will attempt the following:
      - properly perform the French curl exercise.
      - determine a proper starting weight and record it and the repetitions on the workout data card.
   V. DEMONSTRATION AND CRITIQUE
   A. Student demonstration of the triceps extension exercise.
   B. Instructor critique and explanation.
   C. Student demonstration of the dip and L-seat dip exercise.

    D. Instructor critique and explanation of the exercise.

VI. PRACTICAL WORK

    A. Student teams will attempt the following:
- properly perform the triceps extension, dip and L-seat dip exercise.

      a. record all weight and repetitions on data card.
- use remaining class time to properly perform the exercises discussed in previous classes.

VII. STUDY ASSIGNMENT

    A. Strength training misconceptions.

    B. Biceps:
- location.
- primary function during exercise.

    C. Exercises:
- biceps curl.

LESSON 14

   I. QUESTION AND REVIEW PERIOD

  II. LECTURE MATERIAL

    A. Strength training misconceptions:
- muscle bound.
- converting muscle to fat.
- protein supplements.
- spot reducing.
- illogical fears.
- marathon workouts.
- flexibility.
- effects of strength training on women.

    B. Biceps:
- location.
- primary function during exercise.

 III. DEMONSTRATION AND CRITIQUE

    A. Student demonstration of the biceps curl exercise with a barbell.

    B. Instructor critique and explanation.

 IV. PRACTICAL WORK

    A. Student teams should attempt the following:
- properly perform the biceps curl exercise.
- determine a proper starting weight and record weight and reps on the workout data card.

  V. DEMONSTRATION AND CRITIQUE

    A. Student demonstration of the alternate dumbbell curl.

    B. Instructor critique and explanation of the exercise.

    C. Student demonstration of the preacher curl exercise (if preacher bench is available).

    D. Instructor critique and explanation of the exercise.
VI. PRACTICAL WORK
    A. Student teams should attempt the following:
- properly perform the alternate dumbbell curl and the preacher bench curl.
- use remaining class time to properly perform the exercises discussed in previous classes.

VII. STUDY ASSIGNMENT
    A. Review
    B. Exercises:
- wrist curl.
- reverse wrist curl.

LESSON 15

    I. QUESTION AND REVIEW PERIOD
    II. LECTURE MATERIAL
       A. Forearm flexors:
- location.
- primary function during exercise.
       B. Forearm extensors:
- location.
- primary function during exercise.

III. DEMONSTRATION AND CRITIQUE
    A. Student demonstration of the wrist curl exercise.
    B. Instructor critique and explanation.
    C. Student demonstration of the reverse curl and reverse wrist curl.
    D. Instructor critique and explanation of the exercise.

IV. PRACTICAL WORK
    A. Student teams will attempt the following:
- properly perform the wrist curl exercise paying strict attention to execution and proper technique.
  a. record exercise, weight and repetitions on the workout data card.
- use remaining class time to properly perform as many exercises as possible that have been discussed in previous classes.

 V. STUDY ASSIGNMENT
    A. Abdominals:
- location.
- primary function during exercise.
    B. Exercises:
- situp.
- leg raises.

LESSON 16

  I. QUESTION AND REVIEW PERIOD

  II. LECTURE MATERIAL

    A. Abdominals:
- location.
- primary function.

  III. DEMONSTRATION AND CRITIQUE

    A. Student demonstration of the situp exercise.

    B. Instructor critique and explanation of the exercise.

  IV. PRACTICAL WORK

    A. Properly perform the situp exercise.

  V. DEMONSTRATION AND CRITIQUE

    A. Student demonstration of the leg raise exercise.

    B. Instructor critique and explanation of the exercise.

  VI. PRACTICAL WORK

    A. Student teams should attempt the following:
- properly perform the leg raise exercise.
- use remaining class time to properly perform as many exercises as possible that have been discussed in previous classes.

  VII. STUDY ASSIGNMENT

    A. Neck muscles:
- location.
- primary function.

    B. Exercises:
- neck curl.
- neck extension.
- lateral flexion.

LESSON 17

  I. QUESTION AND REVIEW PERIOD

  II. LECTURE MATERIAL

    A. Neck muscles:
- flexors.
- extensors.
- lateral flexors.

    B. Location and primary function during exercise.

    C. Emphasize the importance of developing a very high level of strength in the muscles of the neck (essential for an athlete who plays a sport involving head contact).

  III. DEMONSTRATION AND CRITIQUE

    A. Instructor explanation of the neck curl exercise.

B. Student demonstration of the neck curl exercise with the spotting responsibilities being assumed by the instructor.

IV. PRACTICAL WORK

A. Students will pair off and attempt the following:
- properly perform the neck extension exercise paying strict attention to spotting, execution, and technique.

V. DEMONSTRATION AND CRITIQUE

A. Instructor explanation of the lateral flexion exercise.

B. Student demonstration of the lateral flexion exercise with the spotting responsibilities being assumed by the instructor.

VI. PRACTICAL WORK

A. Remaining class time can be spent performing the exercises discussed in previous classes:
- strict attention must be paid to execution and technique.
- record all exercises, weight, and repetitions on data card.

VII. STUDY ASSIGNMENT

A. Students should prepare and organize a strength development program based on the information they have received in class:
- students should be prepared to discuss their program in the following class.
- attention should be paid to equipment used, number of repetitions executed, number of sets performed, amount of weight used, etc.

LESSON 18

I. QUESTION AND REVIEW PERIOD

II. LECTURE MATERIAL

A. Program organization:
- discussion with the class on how to properly organize a strength development program using the conventional free weight equipment.
- emphasis should be placed on the number of repetitions and sets to be performed, the time interval between exercises, the order of exercises, and the exercises to be performed.
  a. because the student now has a vast inventory of exercises from which to choose, you should organize a few different programs varying the exercises to be performed.

III. A. Review specific exercises that the students are having difficulty with or are not properly performing.

IV. PRACTICAL WORK

A. Student teams will attempt the following:
- properly perform exercises that have been discussed in previous classes.
  a. record all weight and repetitions on data card.

LESSONS 19 & 20

Lessons 19 and 20 can be spent (if facilities allow) performing the specific programs organized by the students.

GRADING

The emphasis placed upon grading will vary with the philosophy of the instructor and the policies of the institution. It should be your goal to determine if your students are capable of independently interacting with all phases of programming, planning, organization, and execution of a strength development program.

The evaluation of your students should be based on criteria you have established for course objectives. Review the practical and cognitive skills that have been established for your course. Include additional objectives to meet the needs of your particular situation. Your evaluation tools should attempt to measure your students' understanding of these particular skills.

Some suggestions on how to grade or evaluate your students include:

• **Class attendance:** As in most other skill-oriented classes, students will not learn the proper skills unless they attend class. A percentage of a student's grade can be based on his/her attendance during the course of instruction.

• **Class participation:** A student's participation during the practical work is mandatory. This is the part of the class in which each student actually lifts weights and experiences the proper execution and techniques which have been advanced by the course. If a student does not actively participate during the exercise portion of the class, he/she will not develop the practical skills needed to perform the exercises properly. A percentage of a student's grade can be the instructor's subjective evaluation of the student's participation during class.

• **Practical skills:** You can evaluate each student's practical application of the information and skills learned in class. This can be accomplished (in a testing situation) by requesting each student to perform a specific exercise and to tell you what he/she is doing so that you know he/she understands the function of the exercise. On the following page is a sample critique sheet you can use for grading. Each student should be required to supplement his/her demonstration with this information.

```
          FRONT                                      BACK

Name:   Mr. Jones

Exercise:   Upright row           Instructor's comments

Muscles used:

Prime mover:

Starting position:

Performance of the exercise:

Spotting:                                    Grade
```

You can also include additional information to meet the demands of your teaching situation. You can grade each specific item or grade the overall performance. A percentage of a student's grade can be based upon his/her demonstration and explanation of the exercise. This particular grading situation can take place anytime during the course of instruction, during the daily student demonstrations, or during scheduled appointments with the instructor other than class time. Near the end of the course, all of the exercises can be written on a piece of paper and placed in a box. Each student can then be requested to select an exercise from all of the exercises discussed in class. This forces your students to be prepared to demonstrate and explain all of the exercises previously discussed in class. This same technique can be utilized with the major muscle groups in the body. You can place the name of each of the major muscle groups into a box and request that each student select a muscle group. That student is then required to prescribe an exercise specific for that muscle group and give the same information listed on the critique sheet above.

• **Cognitive skills:** You can evaluate your students' cognitive skills by periodically administering written exams. A periodic quiz can be administered at the discretion of each instructor. A comprehensive written examination should be given to evaluate each student's understanding of the pertinent material discussed in class. This material should be based on information needed by the student to organize, initiate, and continue a strength development program. Some sample questions include:

1. Which one of the following exercises is usually performed with an **alternate** grip?
   a. upright row
   b. seated row
   c. alternate press
   d. deadlift

2. Which of the following muscle groups are considered the **primary** muscle groups in performing a pullup?
   a. latissimus dorsi, biceps
   b. deltoids, latissimus dorsi
   c. latissimus dorsi, pectorals
   d. deltoids, biceps

3. If you wish to improve your pullup ability which of the following exercises would best meet your objective?
   a. biceps curls, French curls
   b. wrist curls, French curls
   c. lat pulldowns, biceps curls
   d. bent over rows, seated press

Questions 2 and 3 above are designed to determine a student's understanding of the muscles used to perform an activity or exercise, and what exercise should be prescribed to develop those particular muscle groups. Questions of this nature can be designed for all of the exercises and major muscle groups discussed in class. If a student is not capable of understanding this information at the end of your course, he/she will not have the ability to properly organize a functional strength development program. Questions similar to #1 above can be designed to evaluate proper methods and techniques involved in spotting, breathing, and so on.

A question similar to #4 (below) can also be included to evaluate a student's understanding of the exercises that should be performed to develop a specific muscle group.

4. List the core exercise that you would prescribe to strengthen the muscle groups below. The only equipment available is the Universal gym (or the barbell).

   a. quadriceps _____

   b. pectorals _____

   c. triceps _____

Keep in mind that your test questions should attempt to evaluate information needed by your student to organize and understand pertinent concepts of a strength development program. Questions like "Who was Mr. America in 1923?" have no bearing on a student's ability to organize and continue a program upon termination of your course.

If your objectives have been met, you should have a student who is capable of independently organizing a strength development program (based on scientific principles) to improve overall strength. Each student should also be capable of properly executing a multitude of exercises using the most efficient training techniques available.

For an instructor to become competent in the area of strength training, he/she should become very familiar with the basic concepts presented in this book. It would also be to your advantage to initiate and continue a strength development program of your own. This will provide you with a more practical understanding of the training concepts and techniques that are required of effective instructors.

Appendix B

MUSCULAR INVOLVEMENT IN SPORTS

Muscle (corresponds to numbers in Figure B-1.)	Action Numbers in ( ) indicate muscles which assist in action.	Sports In which greatest resistance is encountered
1. Flexor digitorium profundus 2. Flexor digitorium sublimus	Closes fingers	Any sport in which one grasps an opponent, partner or equipment, such as wrestling, hand to hand balancing, tennis, horizontal bar, ball bat, etc.
3. Flexor Pollicis longus	Flexes thumb	
4. Palmaris longus 5. Flexor carpi radialis 6. Flexor carpi ulnaris	Flex wrist palmward and to both sides. (1, 2, 3, 7, 8;	Tennis; throwing baseball; passing a football; handball; ring work; two handed pass in basketball; batting; golf swing.
7. Extensor carpi radialis longus and brevis 8. Extensor carpi ulnaris	Extends wrist	Backhand stroke in tennis and badminton; Olympic weight lifting; bait and fly casting.
9. Pronator teres	Pronates forearm.	Tennis forehand; shot put; throwing a punch; throwing a baseball; passing a football.
10. Supinator	Supination of forearm. (11)	Throwing a curve ball; batting; fencing thrust.
11. Biceps brachii 12. Brachailis	Fexion of elbow. (9)	Ring work; rope climb; archery; pole vaulting; wrestling; back stroke in swimming.
13. Brachioradialis	Strong elbow flexor with forearm pronated or partially pronated.	Rowing; cleaning a barbell; rope climbing.
14. Triceps brachii 15. Anconeus	Extends the elbow.	Breast stroke; shot put; parallel bar work; vaulting; hand shivers in football; hand balancing; batting; pole vaulting; fencing thrust; passing both football or basketball; boxing.

Muscle	Action	Sports Involvement
16. Deltoid. (For simplicity this muscle is divided into anterior and posterior fibers only.)	Anterior fibers—adduction, elevation, inward rotation of humerus. Posterior fibers—abduction, depression, outward rotation of humerus.	Hand balancing; canoeing; shot put; pole vaulting; tennis; archery; batting; fencing thrust; passing a football; tackling; breast stroke; back and crawl strokes; golf swing; handball.
17. Pectoralis major	(A) Forward elevation of humerus. (16) (B) Adduction of humerus. (16, 19) (C) Depression of humerus. (16, 18, 19) Inward rotation of humerus. (18, 19)	Tackling; crawl and back strokes; tennis; passing football; throwing a baseball; javelin; pole vaulting; wrestling; shot put; discus throw; straight arm lever position in gymnastics; punching.
18. Latissimus dorsi 19. Teres major	Draws humerus down and backward. (16) Inward rotation of humerus. (16, 17)	Rope climb; canoe racing; ring work; rowing; batting; crawl, back, breast and butterfly strokes; pole vaulting; golf swing.
20. Trapezius	A. Tilts head back. (23) B. Elevates shoulder point. C. Adducts scapula. (21)	A. Wrestlers' bridge; B. Passing a football; cleaning a barbell; breast stroke. C. Archery; batting; breast stroke.
21. Rhomboids. Major & Minor	Adducts scapula. (20)	Tennis backhand; batting; back and breast strokes.
22. Serratus anterior	Abduction of scapula.	Shot put; discus throw; tennis; archery; tackling; crawl stroke; passing a basketball; passing a football; punching.
23. Spinea erector. (Also includes a number of smaller groups.)	A. Extension of spine. (20) B. Lateral flexion of spine. (20, 26, 27) C. Rotation of spine.	Discus and hammer throw; batting; golf swing; racing start in swimming; diving and tumbling; rowing; blocking in football.
24. External oblique 25. Internal oblique 26. Rectus abdominus 27. Transversalis	Flexion of spine. Lateral flexion of spine. (23) Rotation of the spine. (23) Compression of abdomen.	The importance of this group of muscles in all sports, posture and general fitness and appearance cannot be overstated.
28. Illiopsoas	Flexion of trunk. (27) Flexion of thigh. (36)	Running; hurdling; pole vaulting; kicking a football; line play; flutter kick; pike and tuck positions in tumbling and diving.
29. Sartorius	Flexion of femur. (39) Flexion of knee. Rotates femur outward.	Tumbling and diving.

#	Muscle	Action	Sports
30.	Gluteus maximus	Extends femur. (31, 32, 33) Outward rotation of femur. (31)	Skiing; shot put; running; quick starts in track; all jumping and skipping; line play; skating; swimming start; changing direction while running.
31.	Biceps Femoris	Extension of femur. (30) Flexion of knee. (40) Outward rotation of femur. (30)	Skiing; skating; quick starts in track and swimming; hurdling; line play; all jumping.
32. 33.	Semitendenosus Semimembranosus	Flexion of knee. (40) Flexion of femur. (30) Inward rotation of femur.	
34.	Adductor magnus	Adduction of femur and outward rotation during adduction.	Skiing; skating; frog kick; broken field running; bareback horseback riding.
35.	Gluteus medius	Abduction of femur. (Essential for spring)	Hurdling; fencing; frog kick; shot put; running; line play; skating.
36.	Rectus femoris	Flexion of femur. (28) Extension of knee.	
37. 38. 39.	Vastus internus Vastus intermedius Vastus externus	Extension of knee.	Skiing; skating; quick starts; all jumping; kick in football or soccer; flutter kick; frog kick; water skiing; diving; trampoline and tumbling; bicycling; catching in baseball.
40.	Gastrocnemius	Extension of foot. (44) (when knee is almost straight)	Quick starts in track; swimming; basketball; football; skating; all jumping; skiing.
41.	Soleus	Extension of foot. (when knee is bent)	Changing direction while running; skating; skiing.
42.	Tibialis anterior	Flexes foot and inverts it.	Skating turns; changing direction while running.
43.	Peroneus longus	Extension of foot. (40, 41, 44) Eversion of foot.	Running; all jumping; racing starts.
44.	Flexor hallucis longus	Flexion of big toe. Extension of ankle.	
45.	Sternomastoid	Tucking of chin. Rotation of head. Raises sternum in deep breathing.	Crawl stroke; tucking chin in wrestling, football, boxing; distance running (breathing).

*Reprinted by permission of Cramer Products, Inc.

255

DEFINITION OF ACTIONS

FLEXION — bending at a joint decreasing the angle. Does not apply to shoulder in this chart.

EXTENSION — straightening at a joint, opposite of flexion; not used for shoulder.

ADDUCTION — movement of a part toward the plane which splits the body into two equal halves, left and right.

ABDUCTION — opposite of adduction.

ROTATION — movement of a part around an axis.

PRONATION — rotation of forearm and hand to the palms-down position.

SUPINATION — rotation of forearm and hand to palms-up position; opposite of pronation.

INVERSION — twisting the foot outward at ankle.

EVERSION — bending the foot outward at ankle.

ELEVATION — raising of a part against gravity when in the standing position OR the same movement with the body in other than the standing position.

DEPRESSION — lowering of a part yielding to gravity when in the standing position OR the same movement with the body in other than the standing position; opposite of elevation.

*Reprinted by permission of Cramer Products, Inc.

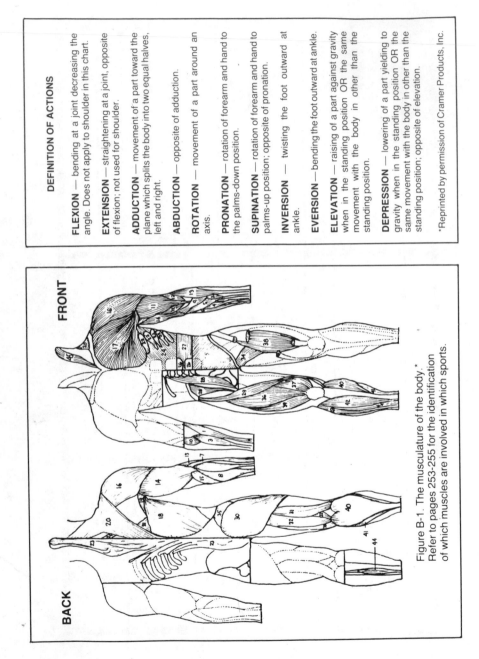

FRONT

BACK

Figure B-1. The musculature of the body.*
Refer to pages 253-255 for the identification
of which muscles are involved in which sports.